CIRCADIAN DIET 2025

110 New Recipes for Weight Loss and Metabolic Wellness Optimize Health Through Meal Timing

KLARLOCK

DISCLAIMER

This book aims to provide useful and informative material on the topics covered in the publication. It is sold with the understanding that the author and publisher are not engaged in rendering any personal medical, health care, or other professional services in the book. The reader should consult his or her physician, health care provider, or other competent professional before adopting any suggestions in this book or drawing any conclusions. The author and publisher expressly disclaim any responsibility for any liability, loss, or risk, personal or otherwise, arising, directly or indirectly, from the use and application of any contents of this book.

NOTE

All the recipes in this book are designed for four people. For this quantity, the ingredients indicated in the recipes must be considered. If you need to change the portion, it is recommended to proportionally adjust the doses of the ingredients. It is also recommended to carefully follow the preparation and cooking instructions to obtain the best result. In the context of this book, when we refer to "a cup" as a unit of measurement for ingredients, we mean using a standard kitchen cup with a capacity of approximately 240 milliliters. It is essential to use a measuring cup to get the right quantities of ingredients. If you don't have a measuring cup, you can use a graduated measuring cup, making sure to correctly correspond to the proportions indicated. Here are some examples 1 Cup of flour 100 gr. 1 cup of rice 200 gr. 1 Cup of Quinoa 200 gr

TABLE OF CONTENT

TASTY APPETIZERS WITH FRUIT

LIGHT AND DIGESTIVE APPETIZERS

RECIPES FIRST DISHES

SOUPS AND STEWS

DISHES BASED ON WHOLE GRAINS

TRADITIONAL DISHES REVISITED

TASTY DISHES WITH FRUIT

DISHES BASED ON TOFU OR SEITAN

229 TOFU SAUTEED WITH VEGETABLES IN THE WOK

231 PAN-FED SEITAN WITH PEPPERS AND ONIONS

233 BAKED TOFU WITH TOMATO AND BASIL SAUCE

235 SEITAN IN SWEET AND SOUR SAUCE WITH BASMATI RICE

DISHES BASED ON LEAN RED MEAT

237 GRILLED BEEF STEAK WITH VEGETABLE SIDE SIDE

239 BEEF STEW WITH SWEET POTATOES

241 PORK FILLET WITH APPLE SAUCE AND CINNAMON

243 ROAST TURKEY WITH AROMATIC HERBS

EGG-BASED DISHES

CREATIVE DISHES

SIDE DISH RECIPES

267 STEAMED VEGETABLES WITH LEMON
YOGURT SAUCE

269 SPINACH SALAD WITH ALMONDS AND
STRAWBERRIES

271 BAKED SWEET POTATOES WITH
AROMATIC HERBS

273 ROASTED CAULIFLOWER WITH
TURMERIC AND PAPRIKA

275 GRILLED COURGETTES WITH BASIL
PESTO

277 SAUTEED GREEN BEANS WITH GARLIC
AND ALMONDS

279 STEAMED ARTICHOKES WITH
MUSTARD SAUCE AND HONEY

281 BAKED TOMATOES WITH BASIL AND
FETA CHEESE

283 SAUTEED MUSHROOMS WITH PARSLEY
AND LEMON

INTRODUCTION TO THE CIRCADIAN DIET

The Circadian Diet Synchronizing Wellbeing with Natural Rhythms Nutrition is one of the crucial elements that influence our health and well-being. Scientific research continues to reveal the importance of not only what we eat, but also when we eat. An innovative and increasingly recognized nutritional approach is the Circadian Diet, a method based on the synchronization of nutrition with the body's natural biological rhythms. Understanding Biological Rhythms Our body follows an internal circadian rhythm, regulated by the biological clock which affects various physiological aspects, including sleep, digestion, metabolism and even mood.

These rhythms are in tune with the natural cycle of sunlight, and the Circadian Diet focuses on how to make the most of these cycles to optimize health. The Importance of Meal Times One of the fundamental pillars of the Circadian Diet is meal times. It's not just about what we eat, but also when we eat it. This nutritional approach suggests concentrating the consumption of more nutritious foods during the daytime, when the metabolism is more active, and reducing the intake of heavy foods during the evening when the body prepares for rest. Key Principles of the Circadian Diet The Circadian Diet promotes a wide variety of natural, unprocessed foods, encouraging the consumption of fruits, vegetables, whole grains, lean proteins, and healthy fats.

It also highlights the importance of reducing consumption of foods high in added sugars, saturated fats and highly processed foods, which can interfere with the body's natural rhythms. The Positive Effects on Health and Wellbeing Following the Circadian Diet could lead to numerous health benefits. Scientific studies suggest that synchronizing nutrition with circadian rhythms can improve metabolism, promote weight loss, increase energy levels and improve the quality of sleep. Furthermore, it may also have positive effects on the immune system and cognitive functions. Your Journey with the Circadian Diet This book is designed to be a practical and comprehensive guide for those wishing to explore the Circadian Diet.

Through delicious and nutritious recipes, balanced meal plans and practical advice, I will take you on a journey to better understand how nutrition can be adapted to your body's natural rhythms. Conclusion The Circadian Diet represents an evolution in the approach to nutrition, inviting us to consider not only what we eat, but also when we do it. This book is designed to offer practical tools and in-depth knowledge to help you reap the full benefits of this approach, leading you towards improved balance and optimal well-being.

THE HISTORY OF THE CIRCADIAN DIET

The history of the circadian diet can be traced back to the mid-20th century, when researchers began studying the human body's circadian rhythm. The circadian rhythm is a 24-hour cycle that regulates many processes in the body, including sleep, digestion, metabolism, and body temperature. In 1971, scientists discovered that light regulates the circadian rhythm. This discovery has led to the development of light-based therapies to treat circadian rhythm disorders, such as jet lag and shift work disorder.

In the 1990s, researchers began studying the impact of diet on the circadian rhythm. They found that eating in harmony with the circadian rhythm can help improve health and well-being.

In 2012, Dr. Satchin Panda, a researcher at the Salk Institute in San Diego, published an article in the journal Science that helped boost the circadian diet. In this article, Dr. Panda demonstrated that eating large meals in the evening can interfere with sleep and increase the risk of obesity and chronic disease. Since then, research on the circadian diet has grown rapidly. Studies have shown that the circadian diet can offer a number of health benefits, including: Improved sleep, Reduced risk of obesity, Reduced risk of chronic diseases, such as type 2 diabetes, heart disease and cancer Improving Cognitive Function, The circadian diet is a relatively new dietary approach, but it is a rapidly growing field of research.

WHAT IS THE CIRCADIAN DIET

The circadian diet is an eating plan that is based on the circadian rhythm of the human body. The circadian rhythm is a 24-hour cycle that regulates many processes in the body, including sleep, digestion, metabolism, and body temperature. The circadian diet suggests that eating in harmony with the circadian rhythm can help improve health and well-being. For example, eating large meals in the evening can interfere with sleep and increase the risk of obesity and chronic disease. Fundamental principles of the circadian diet, The fundamental principles of the circadian diet include:

Avoid eating large meals in the evening.

Focus on foods rich in nutrients and antioxidants.

Avoid processed foods, added sugars and caffeine.

The circadian diet suggests focusing on foods rich in nutrients and antioxidants, including: Fruits and vegetables, Legumes, Whole grains

Fish, Chicken, Nuts and Seeds, The circadian diet is a promising dietary approach that can help improve health and well-being. Here are some of the specific benefits of the circadian diet:

Improved sleep: Eating large meals in the evening can interfere with the production of melatonin, a hormone that helps regulate sleep. The circadian diet, which recommends eating smaller, more frequent meals throughout the day and avoiding large meals in the evening, can help improve the quality of your sleep.

Reduced risk of obesity: Eating large meals in the evening can increase calorie absorption and promote fat storage. The circadian diet, which recommends eating smaller, more frequent meals throughout the day and avoiding large meals in the evening, may help reduce the risk of obesity. Reduced Risk of Chronic Disease: Eating large meals in the evening can increase inflammation, which is a risk factor for many chronic diseases.

THE BENEFITS OF THE CIRCADIAN DIET

Research suggests that the circadian diet may offer a number of health benefits, including:

Improved sleep

Reduced risk of obesity

Reduced risk of chronic diseases, such as type 2 diabetes, heart disease and cancer

Improved cognitive function

Improved sleep

The circadian rhythm regulates the sleep-wake cycle. Eating in harmony with your circadian rhythm can help improve the quality of your sleep. For example, eating large meals in the evening can interfere with the production of melatonin, a hormone that helps regulate sleep.

Reduced risk of obesity

Obesity is a growing public health problem. Research suggests that the circadian diet may help reduce the risk of obesity. For example, eating large meals in the evening can increase calorie absorption and promote fat storage.

Reduced risk of chronic diseases

Chronic diseases, such as type 2 diabetes, heart disease and cancer, are the leading causes of death worldwide. Research suggests that the circadian diet may help reduce the risk of these diseases. For example, eating large meals in the evening can increase inflammation, which is a risk factor for many chronic diseases.

Improved cognitive function

Cognitive function, such as memory and attention, declines with age. Research suggests that the circadian diet may help improve cognitive function. For example, eating large meals in the evening can increase the production of free radicals, which can damage brain cells. How to follow the circadian diet Here are some tips for following the circadian diet: Eat smaller, more frequent meals throughout the day. Avoid eating large meals in the evening. Focus on foods rich in nutrients and antioxidants. Avoid processed foods, added sugars and caffeine. It's important to find a balance that works for you and your lifestyle. If you have questions or concerns, talk to your doctor or a dietitian.

WEIGHT LOSS

The Circadian Diet can be helpful for weight loss. By focusing on eating larger meals during the day and reducing your intake in the evening, you can boost your metabolism and better manage your energy. Additionally, reducing consumption of high-calorie foods and added sugars may be beneficial for weight control. Circadian Diet for Heart Health: The Circadian Diet can support heart health through weight control. Reducing your intake of foods high in saturated fats and added sugars can help reduce the risk of heart disease. Other Specific Applications: Metabolism Regulation: Adapting your diet to circadian rhythms can help regulate your metabolism, supporting energy balance and weight management. Improved Sleep and Rest: A well-structured circadian diet can promote better sleep, as it avoids heavy meals before bedtime and can help regulate sleep-wake cycles. Improved Energy and Attention: Synchronizing nutrition with circadian rhythms can support more stable energy levels throughout the day, promoting greater concentration and attention. Managing Diabetes and Metabolic Health: Adapting your circadian diet can be helpful in managing diabetes and metabolic health, as balancing your meals throughout the day can positively influence blood sugar and insulin levels. Customizing your Circadian Diet to meet specific goals can be beneficial, but it's important to tailor it to your individual needs and consult a health professional, such as a nutritionist or doctor, for personalized advice.

RHYTHM FUNDAMENTALS

The circadian rhythm represents a biological cycle of approximately 24 hours that regulates various physiological processes in the human body and in many other living organisms. These cycles are mainly influenced by variations in sunlight during the day and darkness during the night. Some fundamentals of the circadian rhythm include: Internal Biological Clock: Every individual has an internal biological clock, located primarily in the hypothalamus, which regulates circadian rhythms. This biological clock is influenced by external signals, such as sunlight, that inform the body when it is day and when it is night. Regulation of Physiological Processes: Circadian rhythms influence a wide range of physiological processes, including the sleep-wake cycle, metabolism, digestion, body temperature, blood pressure and hormone secretion. Synchronization with Light and Darkness: Sunlight is the main environmental signal that influences circadian rhythms. Daylight stimulates the body, signaling the start of the day and activating various biological processes, while darkness at night signals the body to prepare for rest. Impact on Health and Wellbeing: The synchronization of circadian rhythms is crucial for overall health and well-being. An alteration of circadian rhythms can negatively affect the quality of sleep, metabolism, mood, concentration and can be associated with health problems such as sleep disorders, obesity, metabolic disorders and other medical conditions. Adaptability and Individual Variations:

Circadian rhythms can vary between individuals, with some people identifying as "early risers" and others as "night owls." Some individuals may be more adapted to certain sleep and wake times than others. Role of Nutrition and Exercise: Nutrition and exercise can also influence circadian rhythms. A diet and exercise regime suited to circadian rhythms can support the body's synchronization and improve overall well-being. Understanding and respecting circadian rhythms can help optimize health, energy and daily productivity, providing helpful guidance for planning daily activities, including sleep, meals and physical activity.

BREAKFAST AND DINNER TIMES

Optimal times for breakfast, lunch and dinner may vary based on individual lifestyle and personal commitments, but here is a general guide for these meals: Breakfast: It is best to eat breakfast within an hour or two of waking up. Eating a nutritious, balanced breakfast early in the morning can help provide energy to start your day and kickstart your metabolism. Lunch: Lunch should be eaten mid-day, around noon or shortly after. This meal should be the largest of the day and include a variety of nutrients to provide energy for the rest of the day. Dinner: It is recommended to consume dinner within the early hours of the evening, preferably at least three hours before going to sleep.

Dinner should be light and composed mainly of easily digestible foods, so as not to disturb sleep or interfere with nighttime digestion. Ideally, these meals should be spaced out in a way that supports the body's natural circadian rhythms, favoring larger meals during the day when the metabolism is most active and reducing food intake during the evening and night. However, it is important to adapt these times to your personal needs, considering work and family commitments and individual preferences. Maintaining a regular mealtime routine can be beneficial in synchronizing your nutrition with your body's natural rhythms.

PHYSICAL EXERCISE

Physical activity plays a crucial role in the context of the circadian rhythm, influencing sleep, metabolism and overall health. Here are some benefits and tips related to physical activity within the circadian rhythm: Benefits of Physical Activity in the Circadian Context: 1. Sleep Regulation: Regular physical activity, especially during the day, can improve the quality of sleep at night , contributing to a deeper and more restful sleep. 2. Circadian Rhythm Synchronization: Exercising throughout the day can help synchronize your internal body clock, contributing to better alignment of circadian rhythms. 3. Metabolism and Weight Control: Physical activity can support metabolism during daytime hours, contributing to weight management and energy balance. 4. Improved Mood and Mental Health:

Regular exercise can promote the production of endorphins, improve mood and reduce stress, contributing to overall well-being. Training Schedule: 1. Morning Exercise: Training in the morning can be beneficial, as it can increase energy levels for the entire day, support concentration and promote regular sleep at night. 2. Moderate Training in the Early Afternoon: Moderate physical activity in the early afternoon can help counteract the natural decline in energy in the early afternoon. 3. Avoid Workouts Too Close to the Evening: Avoid intense workouts in the evening hours as they could overstimulate the body, interfering with sleep. Tips for a Circadian Fitness Regimen: 1. Consistency: Try to maintain a regular physical activity routine, trying to exercise at more or less the same times each day.

2. Variation: Alternating between moderate intensity exercises and more intense workouts can help maintain interest and provide a variety of physical stimulation. **3. Listening to the Body:** Respect your body's signals. If you feel exhausted or too tired, it may be time to take a break or reduce the intensity of your workout. **4. Hydration and Nutrition:** Make sure you drink enough water and eat a balanced diet to support energy and recovery after training. Integrating physical activity in harmony with circadian rhythms can lead to significant benefits for overall health and well-being. However, it is important to adapt physical activity to your needs and consult a fitness professional or doctor before starting a new exercise program, especially if you have pre-existing medical conditions.

COMMON CHALLENGES OF THE CIRCADIAN DIET AND HOW TO OVERCOME THEM

The circadian diet, while beneficial to health and well-being, can present some challenges in its implementation.

1. Changing Eating Habits:

Changing your eating habits to align with your circadian rhythm can take time and effort. It may be difficult to give up foods and drinks you are used to, especially if consumed in the evening or late at night.

How to overcome it:

Start gradually: Don't completely upend your diet in one fell swoop. Introduce changes gradually, starting with small changes like a bigger breakfast or a lighter dinner.

Find healthy alternatives: Replace unhealthy foods and drinks with more nutritious, circadian-friendly alternatives. For example, instead of sweet snacks in the evening, opt for fresh fruit or Greek yogurt.

Plan meals: Planning meals in advance can help you make healthier choices and avoid giving in to temptation when you're hungry.

Cook at home: Cooking at home allows you to control the ingredients and prepare healthier meals that suit your circadian rhythm.

2. Sleep Problems:

The circadian diet aims to synchronize meals with your natural circadian rhythm, which also includes sleep. If you already have sleep problems, lining up your meals may initially make the situation worse.

How to overcome it:

Establish a sleep routine:

Try to go to bed and wake up at the same time every day, even on weekends. This will help regulate your body clock.

Create a sleep-friendly environment: Make sure your bedroom is dark, quiet and cool. Avoid using electronic devices before bed, as the blue light emitted can interfere with the production of melatonin, the sleep hormone.

Practice relaxation techniques: Activities such as yoga, meditation or deep breathing can help you relax before bed.

Avoid caffeine and alcohol in the evening: These substances can interfere with sleep.

3. Flexibility and Adaptation:

Daily life can present unexpected events that make it difficult to strictly follow the circadian diet.

You may need to adjust to work commitments, travel or social events that require you to eat out of hours or consume foods that are not suitable for your diet.

How to overcome it:

Plan ahead: If you know you'll have to eat after hours, try to plan ahead and choose healthier options on the menu.

Bring healthy snacks: If you have the option, bring healthy snacks such as fruits, vegetables or nuts with you to avoid having to resort to unhealthy foods when you feel hungry.

Be gentle with yourself: Don't be discouraged if sometimes you can't follow your diet perfectly. Remember that it's important to do your best and that every little progress is a step in the right direction.

CONCLUSIONS AND NEXT STEPS FOR THE CIRCADIAN DIET

The circadian diet offers a holistic approach to health and wellness, aligning our meals with the body's natural rhythm to optimize energy, sleep, weight loss and overall health. While its implementation may present challenges, the long-term benefits can be significant.

Summary of key points:

Synchronize meals with your circadian rhythm: Eat most of your food during the day, when levels of fat-burning hormones are highest, and have a light dinner.

Choose healthy and nutritious foods: Give priority to fruit, vegetables, whole grains, lean proteins and healthy fats.

Avoid unhealthy foods: Limit sugary, fatty, processed foods, caffeine and alcohol, especially in the evening.

Promote restful sleep: Establish a regular sleep routine, create a sleep-friendly environment, and practice relaxation techniques.

Manage stress: Find healthy ways to deal with stress, such as yoga, meditation, or spending time in nature.

Be flexible and adaptable: Plan ahead for after-hours meals, bring along healthy snacks, and don't be discouraged by occasional lapses.

Seek social support: Talk to friends and family, join a support group, or find a mentor to increase motivation. Next steps:

Do your research: Deepen your knowledge of the circadian diet by reading reputable books, articles, and websites.

Consult a doctor or dietitian: Talking with a health professional can help you evaluate whether the circadian diet is right for you and develop a personalized plan. Start gradually: Don't completely upend your diet in one fell swoop. Introduce changes gradually, starting with small changes.

Listen to your body: Pay attention to how you feel and adjust your diet and habits based on your individual needs.

Be patient and persevere: The circadian diet is a long-term journey. Don't be discouraged if you don't see immediate results. Keep doing your best and you will see the benefits over time.

Remember, the circadian diet is a way to take care of yourself and improve your health and well-being. With hard work and dedication, you can achieve your goals and live a healthier, happier life.

RECIPES APPETIZERS

QUINOA AND FRESH VEGETABLES SALAD

Preparation Times: 15 minutes

Cooking Times: 15 minutes

Doses for 4 People

Ingredients

Quinoa: 200g

Cherry tomatoes: 200g

Cucumbers: 150g

Peppers: 150g

Black olives: 50g

Green olives: 50g

Seasoning to taste

(oil, vinegar, salt, pepper): to taste

Preparation:

Cook the quinoa as directed on the package. Let cool. Cut the cherry tomatoes, cucumbers and peppers into cubes. Combine the chopped vegetables with the cooled quinoa. Add the black and green olives. Season with oil, vinegar, salt and pepper to taste. Mix well and serve fresh.

COURGETTE CARPACCIO WITH AVOCADO SAUCE

Preparation Times: 10 minutes

Cooking Times: None

Doses for 4 People

Ingredients

Courgettes: 300g Avocado: 150g

Lemon juice: 1 lemon

Extra virgin olive oil: 30g

Salt and Pepper To Taste

Preparation:

Thinly slice the courgettes (you can use a mandolin). Blend the avocado with the lemon juice, oil, salt and pepper until you obtain a creamy sauce. Arrange the courgette slices on a serving plate. Pour the avocado sauce over the zucchini. Serve as a fresh and light appetizer.

TOMATO AND CUCUMBER GAZPACHO

Preparation Times: 15 minutes

Cooking Times: None

Doses for 4 People

Ingredients

Ripe tomatoes: 500g

Cucumbers: 300g

Red peppers: 100g

Red onion: 50g

Garlic: 1 clove

Red wine vinegar: 30ml

Extra virgin olive oil: 50ml

Salt and Pepper To Taste

Preparation:

Coarsely chop the tomatoes, cucumbers, peppers, onion and garlic. Blend all the ingredients together (tomatoes, cucumbers, peppers, onion, garlic) until smooth. Add the red wine vinegar, extra virgin olive oil, salt and pepper to taste. Refrigerate for at least an hour before serving. Serve fresh with a basil leaf or croutons.

MELON AND LIGHT RAW HAM

Preparation Times: 10 minutes

Cooking Times: None

Doses for 4 People

Ingredients

Ripe melon: 1

Raw ham: 100g

Fresh mint leaves: to taste 6.

Preparation:

Cut the melon into slices or cubes, depending on your preference. Wrap the melon slices with raw ham. Arrange on a serving plate and garnish with fresh mint leaves. Serve as a fresh and light appetizer, perfect for summer or as a healthy snack.

MUSHROOMS STUFFED WITH AROMATIC HERBS

Preparation Times: 15 minutes

Cooking Times: 25 minutes

Doses for 4 People

Ingredients

Large button mushrooms: 8

Grated bread: 50g

Chopped aromatic herbs

(parsley, thyme, oregano): 20g

Minced garlic: 2 cloves

Grated cheese: 30g

Extra virgin olive oil: 30ml

Salt and Pepper To Taste

Preparation:

Clean the mushrooms and remove the stems. Gently remove the heart of the mushrooms to make room for the filling. In a bowl, mix the breadcrumbs, chopped herbs, garlic, cheese, salt and pepper. Fill each mushroom with the bread and herb mixture. Arrange the mushrooms on a baking tray, drizzle with a drizzle of olive oil and cook in a preheated oven at 180°C for approximately 2025 minutes, until the mushrooms are golden on the surface.

BAKED CAULIFLOWER FRITTERS

Preparation Times: 20 minutes

Cooking Times: 25 minutes

Doses for 4 People

Ingredients

Cauliflower: 1 small

Eggs: 2

Grated cheese: 50g

Flour: 30g

Chopped parsley: 2 tablespoons

Garlic powder: 1 teaspoon

Salt and Pepper To Taste

Extra virgin olive oil: for greasing the pan

Preparation:

Blanch the cauliflower cut into pieces in salted water for 5 minutes. Drain it and let it cool. In a bowl, mash the cauliflower until it has a puree-like consistency. Add the eggs, grated cheese, flour, parsley, garlic powder, salt and pepper. Mix well. Form pancakes with the mixture obtained and place them on a lightly oiled baking tray. Cook in a preheated oven at 200°C for approximately 2025 minutes, until the pancakes are golden and crispy.

RED LENTIL AND GINGER SOUP

Preparation Times: 10 minutes

Cooking Times: 25 minutes

Doses for 4 People

Ingredients

Red lentils: 250g

Onion: 1 medium

Carrot: 1 large

Grated fresh ginger: 2 tablespoons

Garlic: 2 cloves

Vegetable broth: 1 litre

Turmeric powder: 1 teaspoon

Red Chili Powder: 1/2 teaspoon (optional)

Salt and Pepper To Taste

Extra virgin olive oil: 2 tablespoons

Preparation:

Finely chop onion, carrot and garlic. In a large pot, heat the oil and add the chopped vegetables. Cook over medium heat for 5 minutes. Add the red lentils, grated ginger, turmeric and chilli (if using). Stir for a minute. Pour in the vegetable broth and bring to the boil. Reduce the heat and let simmer for about 20 minutes or until the lentils are soft. Blend some of the soup if you want a creamier consistency. Season with salt and pepper, if necessary, and serve hot.

BAKED SWEET POTATOES AL WITH SPICES

Preparation Times: 10 minutes

Cooking times: 25/30 minutes

Doses for 4 People

Ingredients

Sweet potatoes: 4 medium

Extra virgin olive oil: 2 tablespoons

Sweet Paprika: 1 tsp

Cumin powder: 1 teaspoon

Black pepper: 1/2 teaspoon

Salt: to taste 6.

Preparation:

Preheat the oven to 200°C. Wash the sweet potatoes well and cut them into thin slices or cubes. In a bowl, season the sweet potatoes with extra virgin olive oil, sweet paprika, cumin, black pepper and salt. Stir to evenly distribute the spices. Place the sweet potatoes on a baking tray lined with baking paper. Bake in the preheated oven for 2530 minutes, turning the potatoes halfway through cooking, until soft and lightly browned around the edges. Serve hot as a side dish or healthy snack.

SALMON TARTARE WITH AVOCADO

Preparation Times: 15 minutes

Cooking Times: None

Doses for 4 People

Ingredients in grams:

Fresh salmon fillet: 400g

Ripe avocado: 1 large

Lemon juice: 2 tablespoons

Chopped red onion: 1 tbsp

Chopped fresh parsley: 2 tablespoons

Extra virgin olive oil: 2 tablespoons

Salt and Pepper To Taste

Preparation:

Cut the salmon into small cubes and place it in a bowl. Peel and cut the avocado into cubes. Add lemon juice to the avocado to prevent oxidation. Combine the avocado with the salmon. Add the chopped red onion, fresh parsley, extra virgin olive oil, salt and pepper. Gently mix all the ingredients without breaking up the salmon too much. Cover the bowl and let rest in the refrigerator for at least 30 minutes before serving. Serve the salmon tartare on croutons or crackers.

SHRIMP AND CITRUS FRUIT SKEWERS

Preparation Times: 15 minutes

Cooking Times: 57 minutes

Doses for 4 People

Ingredients

Peeled and cleaned prawns: 16

Oranges: 2

Lemons: 2

Extra virgin olive oil: 3 tablespoons

Salt and Pepper To Taste

Preparation:

Cut the oranges and lemons in half and cut into thick slices. Cut each slice into four parts. Thread the prawns onto the skewers alternating them with the citrus fruit segments. Brush the skewers with extra virgin olive oil and season with salt and pepper. Heat a grill or non-stick pan. Cook the skewers for 23 minutes per side or until the shrimp are cooked through and the citrus is lightly caramelized. Serve the hot prawn and citrus skewers as an appetizer or main course, accompanying them with a sauce of your choice.

CROSTINI WITH TUNA AND CAPERS

Preparation Times: 10 minutes

Cooking Times: 57 minutes

Doses for 4 People

Ingredients

Tuna in oil: 200g

Capers: 2 tablespoons

Baguette bread or toast: 8 slices

Extra virgin olive oil: 3 tablespoons

Lemon (juice and grated zest): 1

Chopped fresh parsley: 2 tablespoons

Salt and Pepper To Taste

Preparation:

Drain the tuna from the oil and place it in a bowl. Mash it with a fork. Add the chopped capers, lemon juice, grated lemon zest, fresh parsley, salt and pepper. Mix well. Brush the bread slices with extra virgin olive oil and toast them in a preheated oven at 180°C for about 57 minutes until they are crispy. Spread the tuna and caper mixture on the toasted bread slices. Serve the crostini as an appetizer or snack.

SALMON MARINATED WITH YOGURT AND HERBS

Preparation Times: 15 minutes (more marinating time)

Cooking Times: None

Doses for 4 People

Ingredients

Fresh salmon fillet: 400g

Greek yogurt: 150g

Chopped fresh herbs (parsley, dill, chives): 3 tablespoons

Lemon (juice and grated zest): 1

Salt and Pepper To Taste

Preparation:

Cut the salmon fillet into thin slices. In a bowl, mix Greek yogurt with chopped fresh herbs, lemon juice, grated lemon zest, salt and pepper. Arrange the salmon slices on a plate and sprinkle them evenly with the yogurt marinade. Cover the dish with cling film and leave to marinate in the refrigerator for at least 12 hours. Once marinated, serve the salmon slices on a bed of salad or accompany them with fresh vegetables.

CHICKPEA HUMMUS WITH CRUNCHY VEGETABLES

Preparation Times: 10 minutes

Cooking Times: None

Doses for 4 People

Ingredients

Cooked chickpeas: 400g

Tahini (sesame seed paste): 3 tablespoons

Garlic: 1 clove

Lemon juice: 2 tablespoons

Extra virgin olive oil: 3 tablespoons

Salt and Pepper To Taste

Fresh vegetables of your choice (carrots, celery,

peppers): to accompany

Preparation:

In a blender, place the drained and rinsed chickpeas, tahini, garlic, lemon juice, extra virgin olive oil, salt and pepper. Blend until you obtain a smooth cream. If necessary, add a little water to reach the desired consistency. Cut vegetables (carrots, celery, peppers) into sticks or thin slices to accompany the hummus. Serve the chickpea hummus in a bowl, decorating with a drizzle of oil and accompanying with crunchy vegetables.

BAKED FALAFEL WITH YOGURT SAUCE

Preparation Times: 15 minutes.

Cooking Times: 20/25 minutes.

Doses for 4 People

Ingredients

Cooked chickpeas: 400g

Chopped red onion: 1 small

Minced garlic: 2 cloves

Chopped fresh parsley: 3 tablespoons

Cumin powder: 1 teaspoon

Coriander powder: 1 teaspoon

Paprika: 1 tsp

Chickpea flour: 3 tablespoons

Salt and Pepper To Taste

Greek yogurt: 150g

Lemon juice: 1 tbsp

Chopped fresh mint: 2 tablespoons

Preparation:

In a blender, combine the drained chickpeas, onion, garlic, fresh parsley, cumin, coriander, paprika, chickpea flour, salt and pepper. Blend until you obtain a smooth consistency. With your hands, shape meatballs of similar size and place them on a baking tray lined with baking paper lightly greased with oil. Cook in a preheated oven at 200°C for approximately 2025 minutes, turning the falafel halfway through cooking, until they are golden and crispy. Mix Greek yogurt with lemon juice and chopped mint to make the yogurt sauce. Serve the falafel hot accompanied by the fresh and fragrant yogurt sauce.

BRUSCHETTA WITH DRIED TOMATOES AND PESTO

Preparation Times: 10 minutes

Cooking Times: 57 minutes

Doses for 4 People

Ingredients

Dried tomatoes in oil: 100g

Genoese pesto: 4 tablespoons

Bread (baguette or other

crispy bread): 8 slices

Garlic: 1 clove

Fresh basil for

garnish (optional)

Preparation:

Heat the oven or a grill. Cut the bread into slices and toast them in the oven or on the grill to make it crunchy. Rub a clove of garlic over the bread slices for flavor. Spread the pesto evenly over the toasted bread slices. Cut the dried tomatoes into small pieces and distribute them over the pesto. Garnish with fresh basil leaves, if desired, and serve the bruschetta as an appetizer or snack.

OMELETTE WITH SEASONAL VEGETABLE

Preparation Times: 15 minutes

Cooking times: 15/20 minutes

Doses for 4 People

Ingredients

Eggs: 6

Seasonal vegetables (courgettes,

peppers, tomatoes, spinach, etc.)

approximately 300/400g

Onion: 1 medium

Cheese to taste (parmesan,

pecorino, feta): 50g (optional)

Extra virgin olive oil: 2 tablespoons

Salt and Pepper To Taste

Preparation:

Cut the chosen vegetables into cubes or thin slices and chop the onion. In a non-stick pan, heat the oil and fry the onion with the vegetables until they are well cooked. In a bowl, beat the eggs with salt, pepper and possibly the chosen cheese. Pour the beaten eggs into the pan with the vegetables and cook over medium-low heat until the omelette is set on the edges but still slightly liquid in the centre. If you have a lid, cover the pan for a couple of minutes to cook the surface evenly. Transfer the omelette to a serving plate and cut it into wedges. Serve hot or at room temperature as a main course or accompaniment.

VEGETABLE ROLL WITH GREEK YOGURT SAUCE

Preparation Times: 20 minutes

Cooking Times: 10/15 minutes

Doses for 4 People

Ingredients

Mixed vegetables of your choice (courgettes, peppers, aubergines, carrots): 400g

Brick or phyllo pasta sheets: 8

Greek yogurt: 150g

Chopped fresh mint: 2 tablespoons

Lemon juice: 1 tbsp

Extra virgin olive oil: 2 tablespoons

Salt and Pepper To Taste

Preparation:

Cut the vegetables into sticks or long slices. In a pan, heat a drizzle of oil and cook the vegetables until they are cooked but crunchy. Season with salt and pepper and let them cool slightly. Prepare the rolls: place a portion of vegetables in the center of each sheet of brick or phyllo dough and roll the dough around the vegetables. Place the rolls on a baking tray lined with baking paper and brush them lightly with olive oil. Bake in a preheated oven at 180°C for 1015 minutes or until golden and crispy. In the meantime, prepare the sauce: mix the Greek yogurt with the chopped fresh mint, lemon juice, salt and pepper. Serve the hot vegetable rolls accompanied by the Greek yogurt sauce as a side dish or appetizer.

CRISPY SPICED CHICKPEAS

Preparation Times: 5 minutes

Cooking times: 30/40 minutes

Doses for 4 People

Ingredients

Cooked chickpeas: 400g (rinsed and dried)

Extra virgin olive oil: 2 tablespoons

Paprika: 1 tsp

Cumin powder: 1 teaspoon

Turmeric: 1/2 teaspoon

Salt: 1/2 teaspoon

Black pepper: 1/2 teaspoon

Preparation:

Preheat the oven to 200°C. In a bowl, mix the rinsed and dried chickpeas with extra virgin olive oil, paprika, cumin, turmeric, salt and pepper. Spread the spiced chickpeas on a baking tray lined with baking paper. Cook in the oven for 3040 minutes, stirring occasionally, until the chickpeas are golden and crispy. Let cool slightly before serving. Crispy spiced chickpeas can be a delicious snack or a spicy side dish for main dishes.

GRILLED AUBERGINE ROLLS

Preparation Times: 20 minutes

Cooking Times: 12 minutes

Doses for 4 People

Ingredients

Aubergine: 2 large

Dried tomatoes in oil: 50g

Fresh cheese (ricotta

or anything else to taste): 100g

Fresh basil: 8 leaves

Extra virgin olive oil: 3 tablespoons

Salt and Pepper To Taste

Preparation:

Cut the aubergines into long, thin slices, brush them with olive oil and grill them on a griddle or in a grill pan for 23 minutes per side, until they are soft and well marked by the grill. In a bowl, mix the fresh cheese with the chopped dried tomatoes and a few fresh basil leaves cut into strips. Place some cheese and sun-dried tomato filling on each aubergine slice and roll them up. Secure with a toothpick if necessary. Arrange the rolls on a serving plate, season them with a drizzle of olive oil, salt and pepper, and serve as an appetizer or main course.

CARROT AND HUMMUS SNACKS

Preparation Times: 10 minutes

Cooking Times: None

Doses for 4 People

Ingredients

Carrots: 4 large

Hummus: 200g

Chopped fresh parsley: 2 tablespoons

Toasted sesame seeds

(optional): for garnish

Preparation:

Peel the carrots and cut them into sticks or thin, long slices. Prepare hummus if you don't already have it or use purchased hummus. Prepare the carrot sticks and place them on a serving plate. Accompany the carrot sticks with hummus in a bowl. Sprinkle the hummus with chopped fresh parsley and, if you prefer, add toasted sesame seeds on top to decorate. Serve as appetizers or as part of an assortment of appetizers.

EXOTIC AND INNOVATIVE APPETIZERS

VEGAN SUSHI WITH QUINOA AND VEGETABLES

Preparation Times: 30/40 minutes

Cooking Times: 20/25 minutes

Doses for 4 People

Ingredients

Nori seaweed sheets:

Quinoa: 1 cup

Rice vinegar: 2 tablespoons

Zucchini: 1 large

Carrots: 1 large

Avocado: 1 large

Red pepper: 1/2

Toasted sesame seeds: for garnish

Soy sauce or tamari: for serving (optional)

Preparation:

Cook the quinoa according to the package instructions. Once cooked, season it with rice vinegar and let it cool. Cut the vegetables into long, thin sticks. Place a sheet of nori seaweed on a sushi mat or clean work surface. Spread a thin layer of quinoa over the bottom half of the nori. Place the vegetable sticks and avocado slices on the quinoa. Roll the nori seaweed around the filling using the mat or damp hands, closing the roll tightly. Cut the roll into pieces of approximately 23 centimetres. Garnish with toasted sesame seeds and serve with soy sauce or tamari for dipping.

TOFU AND SEAWEED CROQUETTES

Preparation Times: 20 minutes

Cooking times: 15/20 minutes

Doses for 4 People

Ingredients

Tofu: 400g

Dried seaweed (wakame

or other variety): 30g

Breadcrumbs: 50g

Flour: 3 tablespoons

Onion: 1 medium

Garlic: 2 cloves

Chopped fresh parsley: 2 tablespoons

Extra virgin olive oil: 2 tablespoons

Salt and Pepper To Taste

Preparation:

Soak the dried seaweed in cold water for 1015 minutes, then drain and squeeze them well. Finely chop the onion and garlic. Mash the tofu with a fork or chop it roughly. In a pan, heat the oil and sauté the onion and garlic until golden. Add the seaweed and cook for another 23 minutes. In a bowl, mix the tofu with the seaweed, onion, garlic, parsley, breadcrumbs, flour, salt and pepper. Shape croquettes with your hands and place them on a baking tray lined with lightly oiled baking paper. Cook in a preheated oven at 180°C for approximately 1520 minutes or until the croquettes are golden and crispy. Serve hot as an appetizer or main course.

MIXED VEGETABLE TEMPURA

Preparation Times: 15 minutes

Cooking Times: 10/15 minutes

Doses for 4 People

Ingredients

Mixed vegetables to taste (courgettes, peppers, carrots, onions): approximately 400g

00 flour: 150g

Corn starch: 50g

Ice water: 200ml

Fry oil

salt

Preparation:

Cut the vegetables into sticks or thin slices. In a bowl, mix the flour, cornstarch and a pinch of salt. Add the ice water and mix quickly, leaving the batter lumpy. Heat the oil in a pan or deep fryer to around 180°C. Dip the vegetables in the batter and fry them in hot oil until golden and crispy (about 23 minutes per side). Drain the vegetables on absorbent paper to remove excess oil. Serve the vegetable tempura as an appetizer or main course, accompanying them with soy sauce or other sauces to taste.

STUFFED VINE LEAVE ROLLS

Preparation Times: 30/40 minutes

Cooking Times: 40/50 minutes

Doses for 4 People

Ingredients

Pickled vine leaves

or fresh: 60 leaves

Rice: 250g

Peeled tomatoes: 200g

Onion: 1 large

Chopped fresh parsley: 3 tablespoons

Chopped fresh mint: 2 tablespoons

Lemon juice: 2 tablespoons

Extra virgin olive oil: 4 tablespoons

Salt and Pepper To Taste

Preparation:

If the grape leaves are dry, soak them in water for 30 minutes before using them. Prepare the filling: in a bowl, mix the raw rice, the diced peeled tomatoes, the chopped onion, the parsley, the mint, the lemon juice, 2 tablespoons of oil, salt and pepper. Prepare the rolls: lay out a vine leaf, place a spoonful of filling in the centre, fold the sides inwards and roll up to form a roll. Repeat until you run out of ingredients. Place the rolls in a large pot, overlapping them slightly, and cover them with water. Add another 2 tablespoons of oil and cook over medium-low heat for about 4050 minutes or until the rice is cooked and the leaves are tender. Serve the rolls hot or at room temperature as an appetizer or main course.

BRUSCHETTA WITH FRESH TOMATOES AND BASIL

Preparation Times: 15 minutes

Cooking Times: 57 minutes

Doses for 4 People

Ingredients

Ripe tomatoes: 4 large

Bread (baguette or other bread crunchy): 8 slices

Fresh basil: 1 bunch

Garlic: 2 cloves

Extra virgin olive oil of olive: 4 tablespoons

Salt and pepper:

Preparation:

Cut the tomatoes into cubes and place them in a bowl. Add the chopped fresh basil, salt, pepper and 2 tablespoons of extra virgin olive oil. Mix everything well. Toast the bread slices on a grill or in the oven until crispy. Lightly rub the garlic cloves on the surface of the bread slices. Distribute the seasoned tomatoes on the slices of bread, add a drizzle of extra virgin olive oil and garnish with whole or chopped fresh basil leaves. Serve immediately as an appetizer or snack.

AUBERGINES WITH LIGHT PARMIGIANA

Preparation Times: 30/40 minutes

Cooking Times: 20/25 minutes

Doses for 4 People

Ingredients

Aubergines: 3 large

Peeled tomatoes: 400g

Mozzarella or cheese

vegan to taste: 200g

Grated Parmesan or

vegan alternative: 50g

Fresh basil: 1 bunch

Salt and Pepper To Taste

Extra virgin olive oil: 4 tablespoons

Preparation:

Cut the aubergines into thin slices and grill them on a griddle or in a non-stick pan with a drizzle of oil until they are soft and well marked from cooking. They can also be baked instead of grilled. In a pan, heat two tablespoons of oil and add the peeled tomatoes, salt, pepper and chopped fresh basil. Cook over medium-low heat for about 1015 minutes. On a baking tray, alternate layers of grilled eggplant, tomato sauce, sliced mozzarella (or vegan cheese) and grated parmesan (or vegan alternative), creating multiple layers. Finish with a final layer of tomato sauce and grated parmesan. Bake at 180°C for about 20/25 minutes or until golden on the surface. Let it rest for a few minutes before serving. Serve hot as a main course or light side dish.

BUFFALO MOZZARELLA WITH TOMATOES AND BASIL

Preparation Times: 10 minutes

Cooking Times: None

Doses for 4 People

Ingredients:

Buffalo mozzarella: 2 medium

Cherry tomatoes: 200g

Fresh basil: 1 bunch

Extra virgin olive oil: 4 tablespoons

Salt and Pepper To Taste

Preparation:

Cut the buffalo mozzarella into slices or pieces and arrange them on a serving plate. Cut the cherry tomatoes in half or slices and arrange them around the mozzarella. Chop the fresh basil and sprinkle it over the mozzarella and cherry tomatoes. Season everything with extra virgin olive oil, salt and pepper to taste. Serve as a fresh and light appetizer.

TOMATO AND BUFFALO MOZZARELLA SALAD

Preparation Times: 15 minutes

Cooking Times: None

Doses for 4 People

Ingredients:

Buffalo mozzarella: 2 medium balls

Ripe tomatoes: 4 large

Fresh basil: 1 bunch

Extra virgin olive oil: 4 tablespoons

Balsamic vinegar (optional): 2 tablespoons

Salt and Pepper To Taste

Preparation:

Cut the buffalo mozzarella into slices or cubes and place them in a bowl. Cut the tomatoes into slices or cubes and add them to the bowl with the mozzarella. Chop the fresh basil and add it to the bowl. Season everything with extra virgin olive oil, balsamic vinegar (if used), salt and pepper. Stir gently to evenly distribute the seasonings. Let the salad sit for a few minutes to let the flavors blend. Serve as a fresh side dish or as part of a light appetizer.

WHOLE CROUTTONS WITH FRESH CHEESE AND VEGETABLES

Preparation Times: 15 minutes

Cooking Times: 10 minutes

Doses for 4 People

Ingredients:

Slices of wholemeal bread: 8

Fresh cheese (ricotta, goat's cheese or anything else to taste): 200g

Vegetables to taste (courgettes, peppers, aubergines): 300g

Extra virgin olive oil: 4 tablespoons

Fresh basil: 1 bunch

Salt and Pepper To Taste

Preparation:

Cut the vegetables into thin slices or cubes and grill them on a griddle or in a pan with a drizzle of oil until tender and lightly browned. Toast the slices of wholemeal bread on a grill or in the oven until crispy. Spread the fresh cheese on the toasted bread slices. Arrange the grilled vegetables on top of the fresh cheese. Season with a drizzle of extra virgin olive oil, salt, pepper and fresh basil leaves. Serve as an appetizer or light snack.

SPELLED SALAD WITH GRILLED VEGETABLES

Preparation Times: 15 minutes

Cooking Times: 20/25 minutes

Doses for 4 People

Ingredients:

Spelled: 200g

Vegetables of your choice for grilling (courgettes,

peppers, aubergines): 400g

Cherry tomatoes: 150g

Pitted black olives: 50g

Fresh basil: 1 bunch

Extra virgin olive oil: 4 tablespoons

Balsamic vinegar: 2 tablespoons

Salt and Pepper To Taste

Preparation:

Cook the spelled in boiling salted water following the instructions on the package. Drain it, cool it under running water and leave it aside. Cut the vegetables into slices or cubes and grill them on a griddle or in a pan with a drizzle of oil until they are tender and lightly browned. Cut the cherry tomatoes in half. In a large bowl, combine the cooked farro, grilled vegetables, cherry tomatoes, black olives, hand-torn fresh basil leaves, extra virgin olive oil, balsamic vinegar, salt and pepper. Mix all the ingredients well until they are well seasoned and blended. Let the salad rest for a few minutes before serving. Excellent as a single dish or as a side dish.

WHOLE WHOLE SANDWICHES WITH HUMMUS AND CUCUMBERS

Preparation Times: 10 minutes

Cooking Times: None

Doses for 4 People

Ingredients:

Wholemeal sandwiches: 4

Hummus: 200g

Cucumbers: 2 large

Tomatoes: 2 medium (optional)

Lettuce leaves or

mixed salad: to taste

Preparation:

Cut wholemeal rolls in half. Spread hummus on both inside sides of the sandwiches. Cut the cucumbers into thin slices and, if using tomatoes, cut them into slices too. Arrange the cucumber slices (and tomato, if used) on the bottom of the sandwiches, add lettuce leaves or mixed salad and close with the other half of the sandwiches. Serve immediately as a light snack or quick lunch.

CORN FRIES WITH SPICY SAUCE

Preparation Times: 15 minutes

Cooking Times: 10/15 minutes

Doses for 4 People

Ingredients:

Canned corn: 300g (drained)

Corn flour: 100g

Egg: 1

Onion: 1 small

Chopped fresh parsley: 2 tablespoons

Fresh chilli (optional): 1 small

Salt and Pepper To Taste

Fry oil

Spicy sauce: to serve

Preparation:

Drain the corn and place it in a bowl. Finely chop the onion and chilli (if using) and add to the corn. Add the corn flour, egg, chopped fresh parsley, salt and pepper. Mix the mixture well. Heat plenty of oil in a non-stick pan. Scoop out portions of the corn mixture and place them in the pan, flattening them slightly to form pancakes. Fry them on both sides until golden and crispy (about 34 minutes per side). Drain them on absorbent paper to remove excess oil. Serve the corn fritters hot with spicy sauce on the side, ideal as an appetizer or main course accompanied by a fresh salad.

PINZIMONIO WITH FRUIT SAUCES

Preparation Times: 10/15 minutes

Cooking Times: None

Doses for 4 People

Ingredients:

Raw vegetables to taste (carrots, celery, peppers, cucumbers, cherry tomatoes, etc.):

Fruit sauce (strawberries, blueberries, raspberries, or exotic fruit): 200g

Greek yogurt or light mayonnaise: 150g

Lemon juice: 1 lemon

Salt and Pepper To Taste

Preparation:

Cut raw vegetables (carrots, celery, peppers, cucumbers, etc.) into sticks or pieces for dipping. Make the sauces: In two separate bowls, mix the fruit sauce with half the lemon juice in one bowl and the Greek yogurt or mayonnaise with the other half of the lemon juice in the other bowl. Add salt and pepper if necessary. Arrange the sauces in small bowls and place them on a serving plate along with the chopped raw vegetables. Serve as an appetizer or side dish, dipping the vegetables in the various sauces.

CROSTINI WITH FIGS AND GOAT CHEESE

Preparation Times: 15 minutes

Cooking Times: 57 minutes

Doses for 4 People

Ingredients:

Ripe figs: 8

Goat cheese: 150g

Bread (baguette or other crusty bread): 8 slices

Honey: 2 tablespoons

Chopped Walnuts (optional): 2 tbsp

Fresh rosemary (optional): a few needles

Extra virgin olive oil:

to brush the bread

Preparation:

Cut the figs into thin slices. Cut the goat cheese into slices or pieces. Toast the bread slices on a grill or in the oven until crispy. Lightly brush the bread slices with a little extra virgin olive oil. Place a slice of goat's cheese and a slice of fig on each slice of bread. Sprinkle a drizzle of honey over each crouton and, if desired, add chopped walnuts and a few fresh rosemary needles. Bake at 350°F for about 57 minutes or until the cheese begins to melt. Serve the crostini hot as an appetizer or as a delicious snack.

GUACAMOLE WITH FRUIT CHIPS

Preparation Times: 15 minutes

Cooking Times: 10/15 minutes

Doses for 4 People

Ingredients:

Ripe avocado: 2

Ripe tomatoes: 2 medium

Red onion: 1 small

Fresh coriander: 2 tablespoons (optional)

Lime juice: 1 lime

Salt and Pepper To Taste

Fresh fruit (strawberries, pineapple, mango, etc.): to taste

Preparation:

Peel the avocados and mash them with a fork in a large bowl. Dice the tomatoes and red onion, chop the fresh coriander and add to the avocado. Squeeze the lime juice over the ingredients in the bowl and mix everything well. Season with salt and pepper to taste. To prepare fruit chips, cut fruit (strawberries, pineapple, mango, etc.) into thin slices. Arrange the fruit slices on a baking tray lined with baking paper and cook them in a preheated oven at 120°C for approximately 1015 minutes until they become crispy. Serve guacamole with fruit chips as an appetizer or snack.

POMEGRANATE ARUGULA AND WALNUTS SALAD

Preparation Times: 15 minutes

Cooking Times: None

Doses for 4 People

Ingredients:

Fresh Arugula: 150g

Pomegranate seeds: from 1 pomegranate

Walnuts: 50g

Cheese (feta or other

to taste): 50g (optional)

Balsamic vinegar: 2 tablespoons

Extra virgin olive oil: 2 tablespoons

Salt and Pepper To Taste

Preparation:

Wash and dry the Arugula well and place it in a bowl. Add the previously extracted pomegranate seeds and the coarsely crumbled walnuts. If desired, add shredded cheese. In a separate bowl, mix the balsamic vinegar with the extra virgin olive oil, salt and pepper. Season the Arugula, pomegranate and walnut salad with the vinaigrette prepared just before serving. Mix well and bring to the table as a side dish or light appetizer.

GRILLED VEGETABLES WITH BALSAMIC VINEGAR

Preparation Times: 15 minutes

Cooking Times: 10/15 minutes

Doses for 4 People

Ingredients:

Mixed vegetables (courgettes, aubergines, peppers, onions, etc.): 800g

Balsamic vinegar: 4 tablespoons

Extra virgin olive oil: 4 tablespoons

Salt and pepper:

Preparation:

Cut vegetables (zucchini, eggplant, peppers, onions, etc.) into slices or similarly sized pieces for even cooking. Heat the grill or a non-stick pan and grill the vegetables until soft and lightly browned. You can also use a grill or oven if you prefer. Once ready, arrange the grilled vegetables on a serving plate. In a small bowl, mix the balsamic vinegar with the extra virgin olive oil, salt and pepper. Pour the vinaigrette obtained over the grilled vegetables and mix gently. Serve as a side dish or light main course.

STEAMED VEGETABLE PAN

Preparation Times: 20 minutes

Cooking Times: 30/35 minutes

Doses for 4 People

Ingredients:

Potatoes: 400g

Carrots: 300g

Courgettes: 300g

Peas (fresh or frozen): 200g

Eggs: 3

Grated cheese (parmesan

or anything else to taste): 50g

Milk: 100ml, Butter: 20g

Nutmeg: to taste, Salt and pepper: to taste

Preparation:

Peel the potatoes and carrots, cut them into cubes together with the courgettes. Steam the vegetables until they are tender but not too soft. Cook the peas in boiling water for a few minutes until tender. In a bowl, beat the eggs with the milk, the grated cheese, salt, pepper and a grated nutmeg. Add the cooked vegetables to the egg mixture and mix well. Butter a baking tray and pour in the vegetable mixture. Bake at 180°C for approximately 3035 minutes or until the flan is golden on the surface. Let cool slightly before serving. Excellent as a vegetarian main course or as a side dish.

MARINATED CUCUMBERS WITH YOGURT AND MINT

Preparation Times: 15 minutes

Cooking Times: None

Doses for 4 People

Ingredients:

Cucumbers: 4

Greek yogurt: 200g

Fresh mint: 2 tablespoons finely chopped

Lemon juice: 1 lemon

Garlic: 1 clove (optional)

Extra virgin olive oil: 2 tablespoons

Salt and Pepper To Taste

Preparation:

Cut the cucumbers into thin slices or rounds and place them in a large bowl. In another bowl, mix the Greek yogurt with the chopped fresh mint, lemon juice, minced garlic (if using), extra virgin olive oil, salt and pepper. Pour the yogurt sauce over the cucumbers and mix gently so that they are well coated with the marinade. Cover the bowl with cling film and leave to marinate in the refrigerator for at least 30 minutes. Serve as a starter or fresh side dish.

ROMAN-STYLE ARTICHOKES WITH LEMON AND OIL

Preparation Times: 20 minutes

Cooking times: 30/40 minutes

Doses for 4 People

Ingredients:

Artichokes: 4 large

Lemon: 1

Fresh parsley: 2 tablespoons finely chopped

Garlic: 2 cloves

Extra virgin olive oil: 4 tablespoons

Salt and Pepper To Taste

Preparation:

Clean the artichokes by removing the tough outer leaves, cut off the tips and cut into halves or quarters. Also remove the central hay. Place the artichokes in a bowl with cold water and lemon juice to prevent them from blackening. Drain and dry them well. Place them in a pan with boiling water and cook for about 20 minutes until tender. Drain the artichokes and arrange them on a serving plate. In a bowl, mix the extra virgin olive oil with the lemon juice, chopped garlic, fresh parsley, salt and pepper. Pour the dressing obtained over the artichokes while they are still hot and let them marinate for at least 10 minutes before serving. Excellent as an appetizer or side dish.

RECIPES
FIRST DISHES

LENTIL AND VEGETABLE SOUP

Preparation Times: 15 minutes

Cooking Times: 40 minutes

Doses for 4 People

Ingredients:

Dried lentils: 200g

Celery: 2 stalks

Carrots: 2

Onion: 1

Ripe tomatoes: 2

Vegetable broth: 1.5 litres

Extra virgin olive oil: 2 tablespoons

Fresh parsley: 2 tablespoons finely chopped

Salt and Pepper To Taste

Preparation:

Finely chop celery, carrots, onion and tomatoes. In a large pot, heat the extra virgin olive oil and fry the onion until it becomes transparent. Add celery and carrots, cook for a few minutes, then add the tomatoes and cook briefly. Add the lentils and vegetable broth. Bring to the boil, then reduce the heat and cook over medium-low heat for about 3040 minutes or until the lentils and vegetables are tender. Season with salt and pepper, sprinkle with chopped fresh parsley and serve hot. You can add a splash of extra virgin olive oil before serving.

SPRING MINESTRONE WITH WHOLE GRAINS

Preparation Times: 20 minutes

Cooking times: 30/40 minutes

Doses for 4 People

Ingredients:

Whole grains (spelt, barley, quinoa, etc.): 150g

Courgettes: 2

Carrots: 2

Fresh or frozen peas: 150g

Ripe tomatoes: 2

Onion: 1

Vegetable broth: 1.5 litres

Extra virgin olive oil: 2 tablespoons

Fresh parsley: 2

tablespoons finely chopped

Salt and Pepper To Taste

the preparation:

If using raw whole grains, cook them according to package instructions in boiling salted water. Drain them and leave them aside. Cut the courgettes, carrots, tomatoes and onion into cubes or slices. In a large pot, heat the extra virgin olive oil and fry the onion until it becomes transparent. Add the courgettes, carrots, tomatoes, peas and vegetable broth. Bring to the boil, reduce the heat and cook for approximately 3040 minutes until the vegetables are tender. Add the cooked whole grains to the minestrone, mix well, season with salt and pepper, sprinkle with chopped fresh parsley and serve hot.

CARROT AND GINGER CREAM

Preparation Times: 15 minutes

Cooking times: 25/30 minutes

Doses for 4 People

Ingredients:

Carrots: 500g

Potatoes: 2 medium

Grated fresh ginger: 1 tbsp

Vegetable broth: 1 litre

Onion: 1

Extra virgin olive oil: 2 tablespoons

Salt and Pepper To Taste

Preparation:

Peel the carrots and potatoes, cut them into cubes. Finely chop the onion. In a pan, heat the extra virgin olive oil and fry the onion until it becomes transparent. Add the chopped carrots and potatoes, then add the vegetable broth. Bring to the boil, reduce the heat and cook for approximately 2530 minutes or until the vegetables are soft. Add the grated ginger to the pot and mix well. Blend everything with an immersion blender until you obtain a smooth cream. If necessary, add salt and pepper to taste. Serve hot.

BEAN AND TOMATO SOUP

Preparation Times: 15 minutes

Cooking times: 30/40 minutes

Doses for 4 People

Ingredients:

Cannellini beans: 400g

Ripe tomatoes: 4

Onion: 1

Garlic: 2 cloves

Vegetable broth: 1 litre

Fresh rosemary: 1 sprig

Extra virgin olive oil: 2 tablespoons

Salt and Pepper To Taste

Preparation:

If using dried beans, soak them in cold water for at least 8 hours or according to package instructions. Drain and rinse them. If using canned beans, drain and rinse under running water. Finely chop the onion and garlic. Cut the tomatoes into cubes. In a large pan, heat the extra virgin olive oil and fry the garlic and onion until golden. Add the diced tomatoes, beans and vegetable broth. Also add the fresh rosemary. Bring to the boil, reduce the heat and leave to cook over medium-low heat for approximately 3040 minutes. Add salt and pepper to taste. Serve hot.

WHOLEMEAL RISOTTO WITH MUSHROOMS AND PARSLEY

Preparation Times: 10 minutes

Cooking Times: 35 minutes

Doses for 4 People

Ingredients:

Brown rice: 320g

Mixed mushrooms (porcini, champignons, etc.): 300g

Vegetable broth: 1 litre

Onion: 1

Garlic: 2 cloves

Dry white wine: 120ml

Extra virgin olive oil: 2 tablespoons

Fresh parsley: 3 tablespoons finely chopped,
Salt and pepper: to taste

Preparation:

Clean and cut the mushrooms into thin slices. Finely chop the onion and garlic. In a large pan, heat the extra virgin olive oil and fry the garlic and onion until golden. Add the mushrooms and cook until golden. Add the brown rice and toast it for a couple of minutes, stirring constantly. Deglaze with white wine and let the alcohol evaporate. Gradually add the hot vegetable broth, one ladle at a time, stirring occasionally. Continue cooking for approximately 3035 minutes or until the rice is cooked al dente and has absorbed the broth. When almost cooked, add the chopped fresh parsley and mix well. If you prefer, you can also add grated cheese. Season with salt and pepper to taste and serve hot.

WHOLEMEAL PASTA WITH SPINACH AND WALNUT PESTO

Preparation Times: 15 minutes

Cooking Times: 1012 minutes

Doses for 4 People

Ingredients:

Wholemeal pasta (penne, fusilli, spaghetti, etc.): 320g

Fresh spinach: 150g

Walnuts: 50g

Garlic: 2 cloves

Grated cheese (parmesan or anything else you like): 50g (optional)

Extra virgin olive oil: 4 tablespoons

Salt and pepper:

Preparation:

Boil the spinach in boiling water for a couple of minutes, drain and cool under cold water. In a blender, blend the cooked spinach, walnuts, garlic, grated cheese (if using), extra virgin olive oil, salt and pepper until smooth. Cook the wholemeal pasta in abundant salted water following the instructions on the package, then drain it al dente. In a pan, combine the drained pasta with the spinach and walnut pesto. Sauté everything over medium-low heat to blend the flavors well for a couple of minutes. Serve hot, adding a drizzle of extra virgin olive oil and a sprinkling of grated cheese if you prefer.

VEGETABLE COUSCOUS

Preparation Times: 15 minutes

Cooking Times: 18 minutes

Doses for 4 People

Ingredients:

Couscous: 300g

Courgettes: 2

Peppers: 2

Carrots: 2

Onion: 1

Garlic: 2 cloves

Vegetable broth: 500ml

Extra virgin olive oil: 2 tablespoons

Turmeric powder: 1 teaspoon

Salt and Pepper To Taste

Preparation:

Cut the courgettes, peppers and carrots into cubes. Finely chop the onion and garlic. In a large pan, heat the extra virgin olive oil and fry the onion and garlic until golden. Add the chopped vegetables and cook for a few minutes. Add the vegetable stock, bring to the boil, then add the couscous and turmeric. Cover the pot with a lid, turn off the heat and let it rest for 10 minutes so that the couscous absorbs the broth and swells. Once ready, fluff it with a fork to make it light and airy. Add salt and pepper to taste and serve hot as a main dish or side dish.

QUINOA SAUTÉED WITH COURGETTES AND CHERRY TOMATOES

Preparation Times: 15 minutes

Cooking Times: 15 minutes

Doses for 4 People

Ingredients:

Quinoa: 300g

Courgettes: 2

Cherry tomatoes: 200g

Onion: 1

Garlic: 2 cloves

Fresh parsley:

2 tablespoons finely chopped

Extra virgin olive oil: 2 tablespoons

Lemon juice: 1 lemon

Salt and pepper:

Preparation:

Rinse the quinoa under running water in a fine sieve. Cook the quinoa according to the instructions on the package, then drain it and leave it aside. Cut the courgettes into cubes, cut the cherry tomatoes in half and finely chop the onion and garlic. In a large pan, heat the extra virgin olive oil and fry the onion and garlic until golden. Add the courgettes and cherry tomatoes to the pan and cook until tender. Add the cooked quinoa to the pan with the vegetables, mix well. Season with salt and pepper. Squeeze the lemon juice over the quinoa and vegetables, sprinkle with finely chopped fresh parsley and mix everything well. Serve hot as a main course or side dish.

PASTA AND CHICKPEAS WITH FRESH CHERRY TOMATOES

Preparation Times: 15 minutes

Cooking Times: 20/25 minutes

Doses for 4 People

Ingredients:

Boiled or canned chickpeas: 400g

Cherry tomatoes: 250g

Short pasta (like mezze

pens, fingers, etc.): 320g

Onion: 1 Garlic: 2 cloves

Fresh rosemary: 1 sprig

Fresh chili pepper (optional): to taste

Extra virgin olive oil: 3 tablespoons

Salt and pepper:

Preparation:

Finely chop the onion, garlic and chilli (if using). Cut the cherry tomatoes in half. In a large pot, heat the extra virgin olive oil and fry the onion, garlic and chilli (if using) until golden. Add the cherry tomatoes and fresh rosemary to the pot and cook for about 5 minutes until the cherry tomatoes start to release their juice. Add the chickpeas (rinsed and drained if canned) and about 1 quart of water to the pot. Bring to the boil, then reduce the heat and simmer over medium heat for about 1015 minutes. Add the pasta to the pot and continue cooking until al dente and has absorbed most of the liquid. If necessary, add salt and pepper. Serve hot, possibly with a drizzle of extra virgin olive oil over each portion.

STEWED LENTILS WITH VEGETABLES

Preparation Times: 15 minutes

Cooking times: 30/40 minutes

Doses for 4 People

Ingredients:

Dried lentils: 300g

Carrots: 2

Celery: 2 stalks

Onion: 1

Ripe tomatoes: 2

Vegetable broth or water: 1 litre

Extra virgin olive oil: 2 tablespoons

Bay leaves: 23 leaves

Fresh thyme (optional): 1 sprig

Salt and pepper:

Preparation:

Clean and dice the carrots, celery, onion and tomatoes. In a pan, heat the extra virgin olive oil and fry the onion until it becomes transparent. Add the carrots and celery and cook for a few minutes until tender. Add the chopped tomatoes, lentils, bay leaf, thyme (if using), and vegetable broth or water. Bring to the boil, then reduce the heat and cook over medium-low heat for about 3040 minutes or until the lentils are soft and have absorbed most of the liquid. Season with salt and pepper to taste and serve hot as a main course or side dish.

BLACK BEAN AND CORN SALAD

Preparation Times: 15 minutes

Cooking Times: None

Doses for 4 People

Ingredients:

Black beans (canned, drained): 400g

Sweet corn (canned, drained): 200g

Cherry tomatoes: 250g

Fresh red chili pepper: 1 (optional)

Red onion: 1

Fresh coriander: 3 tablespoons finely chopped

Lime juice: 1 lime

Extra virgin olive oil: 3 tablespoons

Salt and Pepper To Taste

Preparation:

Drain and rinse the black beans and corn under running water. Cut the cherry tomatoes in half and finely chop the red onion. If desired, chop the fresh red chili pepper, removing the seeds to make it less spicy. In a large bowl, combine the black beans, corn, cherry tomatoes, red onion, chili pepper (if using), and chopped fresh cilantro. Season the salad with lime juice, extra virgin olive oil, salt and pepper. Mix all the ingredients well. Leave the salad to rest in the refrigerator for at least 30 minutes before serving to allow the flavors to blend better. Serve cold.

MEDITERRANEAN BEANS PASTA

Preparation Times: 15 minutes

Cooking times: 25/30 minutes

Doses for 4 People

Ingredients:

Cannellini beans (or other variety a

pleasure, boiled or canned): 400g

Short pasta (like ditalini,

half penne, etc.): 320g

Ripe tomatoes: 3

Onion: 1 Garlic: 2 cloves

Fresh rosemary: 1 sprig

Vegetable broth or water: 1 litre

Extra virgin olive oil: 3 tablespoons

Salt and Pepper To Taste

Preparation:

Finely chop the onion and garlic. Cut the tomatoes into cubes. In a large pot, heat the extra virgin olive oil and fry the garlic and onion until golden. Add the chopped tomatoes, cannellini beans and fresh rosemary to the pot. Mix well. Add vegetable broth or water to the pot and bring to a boil. Add the short pasta and cook according to the times indicated on the package or until it is al dente and has absorbed the liquid. If necessary, add salt and pepper. Serve hot, possibly garnishing with a drizzle of extra virgin olive oil over each portion.

COURGETTE AND AUBERGINE LASAGNE

Preparation Times: 30 minutes

Cooking Times: 45/50 minutes

Doses for 4 People

Ingredients:

Courgettes: 3

Eggplant: 2

Pasta for lasagna: 200g

Peeled tomatoes: 400g

Onion: 1

Garlic: 2 cloves

Extra virgin olive oil: 3 tablespoons

Grated cheese (parmesan

or anything else to taste): 100g

Mozzarella: 200g

Fresh basil: 10 leaves

Salt and Pepper To Taste

Preparation:

Cut the courgettes and aubergines into long, thin slices lengthwise. In a non-stick pan, grill the courgette and aubergine slices until soft. Set aside. Finely chop the onion and garlic. In a pan, heat the extra virgin olive oil and fry the onion and garlic until golden. Add the peeled tomatoes and basil, season with salt and pepper and cook for 1015 minutes over medium-low heat. Preheat the oven to 180°C.

In a baking pan, start assembling the lasagna by alternating layers of courgettes, aubergines, lasagna pasta, tomato sauce and grated cheese. Continue until you run out of ingredients, making sure the last layer is sauce and cheese. Cut the mozzarella into cubes and distribute it over the grated cheese. Cover the pan with foil and bake for approximately 3035 minutes. Remove the foil and cook for another 1520 minutes until the surface is golden. Let it rest for a few minutes before serving.

COURGETTE SPAGHETTI WITH AVOCADO PESTO

Preparation Times: 15 minutes

Cooking Times: None

Doses for 4 People

Ingredients:

Courgettes: 4

Ripe avocado: 1

Fresh basil: 20 leaves

Walnuts or pine nuts: 50g

Lemon juice: 1 lemon

Garlic: 1 clove

Extra virgin olive oil: 4 tablespoons

Salt and Pepper To Taste

Preparation:

Using a spiralizer or potato peeler, create zucchini spaghetti. Set aside. In a blender, combine the avocado, basil, walnuts or pine nuts, lemon juice, garlic, extra virgin olive oil, salt and pepper. Blend the ingredients until smooth, adding more oil if necessary. In a large skillet, heat the zucchini noodles over medium heat for about 23 minutes without overcooking. Add the avocado pesto, mix well and cook for a further 12 minutes until the spaghetti is well seasoned. Serve hot.

PEPPERS STUFFED WITH RICE AND VEGETABLES

Preparation Times: 30 minutes

Cooking Times: 40/45 minutes

Doses for 4 People

Ingredients:

Large peppers: 4

Brown rice: 200g

Courgettes: 2

Carrots: 2

Onion: 1

Garlic: 2 cloves

Ripe tomatoes: 2

Fresh parsley: 3

tablespoons finely chopped

Extra virgin olive oil: 4 tablespoons

Grated cheese (to taste): 50g

Salt and Pepper To Taste

Preparation:

Cut off the tops of the peppers (like a cap) and remove the seeds and internal strings. Set aside. Cook brown rice according to package instructions. Cut the courgettes, carrots, onion and tomatoes into small cubes. In a pan, heat the extra virgin olive oil and fry the onion and garlic until golden. Add the courgettes, carrots and tomatoes to the pan and cook for about 1015 minutes or until the vegetables are soft.

Combine the cooked rice with the vegetables, add the chopped fresh parsley, grated cheese (if using), salt and pepper. Mix everything well. Fill the peppers with the rice and vegetable mixture. Place the peppers in a baking pan, cover with the previously cut "caps" and bake at 180°C for 4045 minutes until the peppers are soft and lightly golden on the surface.

BAKED POTATOES WITH SPINACH AND CHEESE

Preparation Times: 20 minutes

Cooking Times: 40/45 minutes

Doses for 4 People

Ingredients:

Large potatoes: 4

Fresh spinach: 300g

Grated cheese (parmesan,

pecorino or anything else to taste): 100g

Garlic: 2 cloves

Extra virgin olive oil: 3 tablespoons

Butter: 2 tablespoons

Salt and Pepper To Taste

Preparation:

Preheat the oven to 200°C. Wash the potatoes well, dry them and make deep cuts on the surface. Cook the whole potatoes in the oven for about 40/45 minutes or until they are soft inside and the skin is crunchy. In the meantime, in a pan, heat the extra virgin olive oil and brown the finely chopped garlic. Add fresh spinach and cook until wilted. Salt and pepper to taste. Once cooked, cut the potatoes in half and with the help of a spoon remove part of the internal pulp, placing it in a bowl. Mix the potato pulp with the spinach, grated cheese and butter. Fill the half potatoes with the mixture obtained. Place the stuffed potatoes back in the pan and cook in a preheated oven at 180°C for approximately 15/20 minutes or until the cheese is melted and lightly golden on the surface. Serve hot.

WHOLEMEAL SPAGHETTI WITH CLAMS

Preparation Times: 15 minutes

Cooking times: 15/20 minutes

Doses for 4 People

Ingredients:

Wholemeal spaghetti: 400g

Shelled clams: 500g

Garlic: 3 cloves

Fresh parsley: 4

tablespoons finely chopped

Fresh chili pepper (optional): 1

Dry white wine: 120ml

Extra virgin olive oil: 4 tablespoons

Salt to taste

Preparation:

Bring a pot of salted water to a boil to cook the whole-wheat spaghetti according to the package instructions. In a large skillet, heat the extra virgin olive oil over medium-low heat. Add the chopped garlic and, if desired, the fresh chilli cut into thin slices and fry until the garlic is golden. Add the shelled clams to the pan and deglaze with the white wine. Cover with a lid and cook over medium heat until the clams open. Drain the wholemeal spaghetti al dente, reserving a little of the cooking water. Add the spaghetti to the clams in the pan and add the chopped fresh parsley. Mix well and, if necessary, add a little pasta cooking water to mix everything together. Serve hot with a drizzle of extra virgin olive oil and fresh parsley to decorate.

SALMON FILLET BAKED IN FOIL WITH VEGETABLES

Preparation Times: 20 minutes

Cooking Times: 20/25 minutes

Doses for 4 People

Ingredients:

Salmon fillets:

4 (approximately 150g each)

Courgettes: 2

Tomatoes: 4

Lemon: 1

Fresh rosemary: 4 sprigs

Fresh parsley: 4 tablespoons finely chopped

Salt and Pepper To Taste

Baking paper or aluminum sheets: 4

Preparation:

Preheat the oven to 200°C. Cut the courgettes into rounds and the tomatoes and lemon into thin slices. Cut four sheets of baking paper or aluminum foil (one for each salmon fillet). Arrange a bed of courgettes and tomatoes on each sheet of baking paper or aluminum foil. Place a salmon fillet on top of each bed. Season the salmon fillets with salt, pepper, chopped fresh parsley and fresh rosemary. Add lemon slices on top. Close the parcels carefully, forming pockets, and place them on a baking tray. Bake the parcels with the salmon for about 20/25 minutes or until the salmon is cooked to the desired point. Serve hot directly in foil to preserve flavor and softness.

WHITE BEAN TUNA SALAD

Preparation Times: 15 minutes

Cooking Times: None

Doses for 4 People

Ingredients:

Tuna in oil (drained): 250g

White beans (boiled or

canned, drained): 400g

Cherry tomatoes: 200g

Red onion: 1

Black olives: 50g

Fresh parsley: 3 tablespoons

finely chopped

Extra virgin olive oil: 3 tablespoons

Lemon juice: 1 lemon

Salt and Pepper To Taste

Preparation:

Cut the cherry tomatoes in half and finely chop the red onion. In a large bowl, combine the drained tuna in oil, drained white beans, cherry tomatoes, red onion, black olives and chopped fresh parsley. Season the salad with extra virgin olive oil, lemon juice, salt and pepper. Mix all the ingredients well. Let the salad rest in the refrigerator for at least 30 minutes before serving to allow the flavors to blend better. Serve cold.

RISOTTO WITH SHRIMPS AND COURGETTES

Preparation Times: 10 minutes

Cooking Times: 20/25 minutes

Doses for 4 People

Ingredients:

Arborio or Carnaroli rice: 320g

Shelled shrimp: 300g

Courgettes: 2

Onion: 1

Vegetable broth: 1.5 litres

Dry white wine: 120ml

Butter: 50g

Extra virgin olive oil: 2 tablespoons

Grated cheese (parmesan

or anything else to taste): 50g Salt and pepper: to taste

Preparation:

Heat the vegetable broth in a saucepan and keep it warm over low heat. In a large pan, heat the extra virgin olive oil and add the chopped onion. Sauté the onion over medium heat. Add the rice and toast for a couple of minutes until translucent. Deglaze with white wine and let the alcohol evaporate. Add the courgettes cut into small cubes and the peeled prawns to the pot. Mix well. Gradually add the hot broth, one ladle at a time, stirring constantly and waiting for it to be absorbed before adding more. Continue cooking the risotto for 18/20 minutes, tasting to check the cooking of the rice. When the rice is al dente, remove from the heat and stir in the butter and grated cheese. Adjust salt and pepper according to taste. Serve hot.

VEGETARIAN PAD THAI WITH TOFU

Preparation Times: 20 minutes

Cooking Times: 15 minutes

Doses for 4 People

Ingredients:

Rice noodles: 300g

Tofu: 300g

Red onion: 1

Carrots: 2

Courgettes: 2

Soya sprouts: 100g

Chopped peanuts: 50g

Soy sauce: 4 tablespoons

Lime juice: 2 limes

Brown sugar: 2 tablespoons

Sesame oil: 2 tablespoons

Vegetable oil: 3 tablespoons

Salt and Pepper To Taste

Preparation:

Prepare the rice noodles according to the package instructions. Cut the tofu into cubes and sauté in a pan with a little vegetable oil until golden. Set aside. In a large pan, heat the sesame oil and fry the finely sliced red onion, julienned carrots and courgettes. Add the bean sprouts and egg (if using), stirring well to cook the egg. Add the previously cooked rice noodles, sautéed tofu, soy sauce, lime juice and brown sugar. Continue stirring until all ingredients are well combined and heated through. Serve the Pad Thai hot, sprinkled with chopped peanuts and garnished with lime wedges.

SEITAN SAUTEED WITH CRUNCHY VEGETABLES

Preparation Times: 15 minutes

Cooking Times: 15 minutes

Doses for 4 People

Ingredients:

Seitan: 400g

Peppers (various colors): 2

Courgettes: 2

Onion: 1

Soy sauce: 4 tablespoons

Garlic: 2 cloves

Grated fresh ginger: 1 tbsp

Vegetable oil: 3 tablespoons

Sesame seeds: 1 tbsp

Salt and Pepper To Taste

Preparation:

Cut the seitan into thin slices. Cut the peppers, courgettes and onion into julienne strips. In a large skillet, heat the vegetable oil and fry the minced garlic and grated ginger until golden. Add the seitan and sauté for a few minutes. Add the onion, peppers and courgettes, mixing well. Add the soy sauce and continue sautéing over high heat until the vegetables are crisp but tender. Before serving, sprinkle with sesame seeds. Serve hot.

BAKED SEITAN AND PEPPERS SKEWERS

Preparation Times: 20 minutes

Cooking times: 15/20 minutes

Doses for 4 People

Ingredients:

Seitan: 400g

Peppers (various colors): 2

Onion: 1

Extra virgin olive oil: 3 tablespoons

Lemon juice: 2 tablespoons

Dried oregano: 1 teaspoon

Salt and Pepper To Taste

Skewer sticks (previously

soaked in water to prevent burning)

Preparation:

Cut the seitan into cubes and the peppers and onion into large pieces. In a bowl, mix the extra virgin olive oil, lemon juice, oregano, salt and pepper. Thread the seitan, pepper and onion cubes alternately onto the skewer sticks. Arrange the skewers on a baking tray and brush the previously prepared marinade on all the skewers. Cook in a preheated oven at 200°C for 15/20 minutes or until the seitan and vegetables are golden brown. Serve hot.

TOFU IN TERIYAKI SAUCE WITH BASMATI RICE

Preparation Times: 15 minutes

Cooking Times: 30 minutes

Doses for 4 People

Ingredients:

Tofu: 400g

Basmati rice: 300g

Teriyaki sauce: 120ml

Garlic: 2 cloves

Vegetable oil: 2 tablespoons

Shallot: 1

Sesame seeds: 1 tbsp

Fresh parsley: 2 tablespoons

finely chopped, Salt and pepper: to taste

Preparation:

Cut the tofu into cubes and drain the tofu to remove excess water. In a pan, heat the vegetable oil and fry the minced garlic and thinly sliced shallots until golden. Add the tofu to the pan and cook until golden brown on all sides. Add the teriyaki sauce to the tofu and continue to cook for a few minutes until the tofu is well coated in the sauce. Meanwhile, cook the basmati rice according to the package instructions. Serve the tofu in hot teriyaki sauce, sprinkled with sesame seeds and chopped parsley, accompanied by cooked basmati rice.

MIXED VEGETABLE CURRY WITH BASMATI RICE

Preparation Times: 20 minutes

Cooking Times: 30 minutes

Doses for 4 People

Ingredients:

Basmati rice: 300g

Mixed vegetables (courgettes, carrots, peppers, cauliflower, etc.): 500g

Onion: 1

Garlic: 2 cloves

Fresh ginger grated: 1 tbsp

Coconut milk: 400ml

Curry powder: 2 tbsp

Vegetable oil: 2 tablespoons

Cumin seeds: 1 tsp

Fresh parsley: 2 tablespoons finely chopped

Salt and Pepper To Taste

Preparation:

Cook the basmati rice according to the package instructions. Cut the vegetables into cubes or slices, the onion into thin slices and mince the garlic. In a large pot, heat the vegetable oil and add the cumin seeds, garlic, ginger and onion. Fry until golden. Add the vegetables and cook for a few minutes until they start to soften.

Add the curry powder, mix well and pour in the coconut milk. Bring to the boil, then reduce the heat and leave to cook over medium heat for about 15/20 minutes or until the vegetables are cooked. Adjust salt and pepper according to taste. Serve the mixed vegetable curry hot, accompanied by cooked basmati rice.

SUSHI BOWL WITH SALMON AVOCADO

Preparation Times: 25 minutes

Cooking Times: None

Doses for 4 People

Ingredients:

Sushi Rice or Short Grain Rice: 300g

Fresh salmon (raw): 300g

Ripe avocado: 2

Nori seaweed cut into thin strips: 4 sheets

Soy sauce: 4 tablespoons

Rice vinegar: 2 tablespoons

Toasted sesame seeds: 2 tablespoons

Dried Wakame seaweed (optional): 50g

Preparation:

Cook the sushi rice according to the package instructions. Once ready, add the rice vinegar and mix well. Cut the salmon into cubes and the avocado into slices. Distribute the rice on serving plates and arrange the diced raw salmon, sliced avocado and strips of nori seaweed on top. If desired, add dried wakame seaweed. Sprinkle with toasted sesame seeds and serve with soy sauce on the side for those who wish to further season the dish.

CHINESE-STYLE VEGETABLE STIR-FRY

Preparation Times: 15 minutes

Cooking Times: 10/15 minutes

Doses for 4 People

Ingredients:

Broccoli: 200g

Mushrooms (champignon or shiitake): 200g

Peppers (various colors): 2

Carrots: 2 Onion: 1

Soy sauce: 4 tablespoons

Grated fresh ginger: 1 tbsp

Garlic: 2 cloves

Sesame oil: 2 tablespoons

Vegetable oil: 2 tablespoons

Sesame seeds: 1 tbsp

Salt and Pepper To Taste

Preparation:

Cut vegetables (broccoli, mushrooms, peppers, carrots and onion) into pieces or slices according to your taste. In a large skillet or wok, heat the vegetable oil and add the minced garlic and grated fresh ginger. Fry until golden brown. Add the chopped vegetables and mix well. Add the soy sauce and continue to cook over high heat for 10/15 minutes, stirring occasionally, until the vegetables are cooked but remain crunchy. When almost cooked, add the sesame oil and sesame seeds. Adjust salt and pepper according to taste. Serve the Chinese-style vegetables hot as a side dish or main course.

QUINOA AND VEGETABLES WOK

Preparation Times: 15 minutes

Cooking times: 15/20 minutes

Doses for 4 People

Ingredients:

Quinoa: 300g

Peppers (various colors): 2

Courgettes: 2

Onion: 1

Carrots: 2

Soy sauce: 4 tablespoons

Sesame oil: 2 tablespoons

Garlic: 2 cloves

Grated fresh ginger: 1 tbsp

Vegetable oil: 2 tablespoons

Sesame seeds: 1 tbsp

Salt and Pepper To Taste

Preparation:

Prepare the quinoa following the instructions on the package. Cut the vegetables (peppers, courgettes, onion and carrots) into pieces or slices. In a wok or large skillet, heat the vegetable oil and add the minced garlic and grated fresh ginger. Fry until golden brown. Add the chopped vegetables and mix well. Add the soy sauce and continue to cook over high heat for 10/15 minutes, stirring occasionally. Add the cooked quinoa to the wok with the vegetables, mix well and cook for another 5 minutes. When almost cooked, add the sesame oil and sesame seeds. Adjust salt and pepper according to taste. Serve the quinoa and vegetable wok hot as a main course or side dish.

WHOLEMEAL PASTA SALAD WITH DRIED TOMATOES

Preparation Times: 15 minutes

Cooking Times: 10/12 minutes

Doses for 4 People

Ingredients:

Wholemeal Pasta to taste: 400g

Dried tomatoes: 100g

Fresh rocket: 100g

Pitted black olives: 50g

Feta cheese: 100g

Extra virgin olive oil: 3 tablespoons

Balsamic vinegar: 2 tablespoons

Fresh basil: 1 bunch

Salt and Pepper To Taste

Preparation:

Cook wholemeal pasta in boiling salted water following the instructions on the package. Drain it al dente and let it cool. Cut the dried tomatoes into small pieces and chop the black olives. Also chop the fresh basil. In a large bowl, combine whole-wheat pasta, sun-dried tomatoes, black olives, fresh arugula and basil. Crumble the feta cheese on top. Prepare the vinaigrette by mixing the extra virgin olive oil, balsamic vinegar, salt and pepper. Pour the vinaigrette over the pasta salad and mix well. Serve cold.

SPELLED WITH GRILLED VEGETABLES AND FETA

Preparation Times: 15 minutes

Cooking Times: 20/25 minutes

Doses for 4 People

Ingredients:

Spelled: 300g

Peppers (various colors): 2

Courgettes: 2

Eggplant: 1 Onion: 1

Feta cheese: 100g

Extra virgin olive oil: 3 tablespoons

Balsamic vinegar: 2 tablespoons

Fresh parsley: 2 tablespoons finely chopped

Salt and Pepper To Taste

Preparation:

Cook the spelled in boiling salted water following the instructions on the package. Drain it al dente and let it cool. Slice the vegetables (peppers, courgettes, aubergines and onion). Heat a grill or nonstick pan and grill the vegetables until well cooked and grilled. In a bowl, combine the cooked spelled, grilled vegetables and chopped fresh parsley. Crumble the feta cheese on top. Prepare the vinaigrette by mixing the extra virgin olive oil, balsamic vinegar, salt and pepper. Pour the vinaigrette over the spelled and grilled vegetables and mix well. Serve hot or cold depending on taste.

WILD RICE SALAD WITH CRUNCHY VEGETABLES

Preparation Times: 20 minutes

Cooking Times: 20/25 minutes

Doses for 4 People

Ingredients:

Wild Rice: 300g

Peppers (various colors): 2

Courgettes: 2

Carrots: 2

Onion: 1

Flaked almonds: 50g

Extra virgin olive oil: 3 tablespoons

Apple cider vinegar: 2 tablespoons

Fresh basil: 1 bunch

Fresh mint: 1 bunch

Salt and Pepper To Taste

Preparation:

Cook wild rice in boiling salted water according to package instructions. Drain it al dente and let it cool. Cut the vegetables (peppers, courgettes, carrots and onion) into cubes. In a pan, heat a little extra virgin olive oil and sauté the diced vegetables until they become crispy but tender. Add the flaked almonds and mix well. In a large bowl, combine the cooled wild rice with the crisp vegetables. Prepare the vinaigrette by mixing the extra virgin olive oil, apple cider vinegar, chopped fresh basil and fresh mint, salt and pepper. Pour the vinaigrette over the rice and vegetable salad and mix well. Serve cold.

COLD SPAGHETTI WITH BASIL PESTO

Preparation Times: 15 minutes

Cooking Times: 10/12 minutes

Doses for 4 People

Ingredients:

Spaghetti: 400g

Fresh basil: 1 bunch

Almonds or pine nuts: 50g

Grated parmesan: 50g

Garlic: 2 cloves

Extra virgin olive oil: 4 tablespoons

Salt and Pepper To Taste

Preparation:

Cook the spaghetti in boiling salted water following the instructions on the package. Drain them al dente and let them cool. Prepare the basil pesto by blending together the fresh basil leaves, almonds or pine nuts, grated cheese, garlic, extra virgin olive oil, salt and pepper. Pour the prepared pesto over the cooled spaghetti and mix well until the spaghetti is well seasoned with the pesto. You can add a few whole fresh basil leaves as decoration before serving. Serve cold.

PENNE ALL'ARRABBIATA WITH FRESH TOMATOES

Preparation Times: 10 minutes

Cooking Times: 10/12 minutes

Doses for 4 People

Ingredients:

Penne rigate: 400g

Ripe tomatoes: 4

Fresh chili pepper: 1

Garlic: 2 cloves

Extra virgin olive oil

of olive: 4 tablespoons

Fresh parsley: 2 tablespoons

finely chopped, Salt: to taste

Preparation:

Cook the penne in plenty of salted water following the instructions on the package. Drain them al dente and set them aside. Cut the tomatoes into cubes and chop the chilli and garlic finely. In a pan, heat the extra virgin olive oil and add the chopped garlic and chilli pepper. Let it fry for a minute on medium heat. Add the diced tomatoes to the pan with the garlic and chili pepper. Cook for about 5/7 minutes until the tomatoes break down slightly and the sauce becomes thick. Add the penne to the pan with the prepared sauce, mix well to flavor them and add the chopped parsley. Serve hot, possibly adding more fresh chilli or parsley as decoration.

RICE PILAF WITH SEASONAL VEGETABLES

Preparation Times: 15 minutes

Cooking times: 15/20 minutes

Doses for 4 People

Ingredients:

Basmati Rice or Long Grain Rice: 300g

Seasonal vegetables (courgettes, peppers, carrots, peas, etc.): 400g

Onion: 1

Vegetable broth: 600ml

Butter or extra virgin olive oil of olive: 2 tablespoons

Salt and Pepper To Taste

Preparation:

Cut vegetables (courgettes, peppers, carrots, etc.) into cubes or slices. Finely chop the onion. In a saucepan, heat the butter or extra virgin olive oil and fry the onion until translucent. Add the chopped vegetables to the pot with the onion and cook for a few minutes until tender but crisp. Add the rice to the pot with the vegetables and mix well to combine the flavours. Pour the hot vegetable broth into the pan, bring to the boil and lower the heat. Cover the pot with a lid and let it cook for 15/20 minutes until the rice is cooked and absorbs all the broth. Adjust salt and pepper according to taste. Serve hot as a side dish or main course.

VEGETARIAN LASAGNA WITH LIGHT BÉCHAMEL

Preparation Times: 30 minutes

Cooking Times: 40/45 minutes

Doses for 4 People

Ingredients:

Lasagne sheets: 250g

Courgettes: 2

Eggplant: 1

Peppers (various colors): 2

Mushrooms (champignons or others): 200g

Peeled tomatoes: 400g Onion: 1

Garlic: 2 cloves

Extra virgin olive oil: 3 tablespoons

Grated cheese: 100g

Skimmed milk: 500ml

Flour: 50g

Butter: 50g

Nutmeg: to taste

Salt and Pepper To Taste

Preparation:

Cut vegetables (courgettes, aubergines, peppers and mushrooms) into slices or cubes. In a pan, heat the extra virgin olive oil and fry the finely chopped garlic and onion. Add the chopped vegetables and cook until soft. Add the peeled tomatoes, season with salt and pepper and cook for about 10/15 minutes over medium heat, until the vegetables are cooked and the sauce is thick.

Prepare the béchamel sauce: melt the butter in a pan, add the flour and mix, then pour in the milk little by little, stirring constantly. Cook over low heat until you obtain a creamy consistency. Add some grated nutmeg, salt and pepper. In a baking dish, alternate layers of lasagna pasta, vegetables and bechamel. Finish with a layer of béchamel sauce and sprinkle the surface with grated cheese. Bake at 180°C for approximately 3035 minutes or until the surface is golden. Let it rest for a few minutes before serving.

WHOLEMEAL SPAGHETTI WITH TOMATO AND BASIL

Preparation Times: 15 minutes

Cooking Times: 10/12 minutes

Doses for 4 People

Ingredients:

Wholemeal Spaghetti: 400g

Ripe tomatoes: 6

Garlic: 2 cloves

Fresh basil: 1 bunch

Extra virgin olive oil

of olive: 4 tablespoons

Salt to taste

Preparation:

Cook wholemeal spaghetti in boiling salted water following the instructions on the package. Drain them al dente and set them aside. Peel and mince the garlic. Cut the tomatoes into cubes and chop the fresh basil. In a pan, heat the extra virgin olive oil and fry the garlic until golden. Add the chopped tomatoes and cook over medium heat for 10/15 minutes until you obtain a thick sauce. Add the chopped basil and season with salt. Add the spaghetti to the prepared sauce, mix well and serve hot with a few fresh basil leaves as decoration.

RISOTTO WITH STRAWBERRIES AND FRESH THYME

Preparation Times: 10 minutes

Cooking Times: 20/25 minutes

Doses for 4 People

Ingredients:

Arborio rice: 300g

Ripe strawberries: 250g

Onion: 1

Vegetable broth: 1L

Dry white wine: 120ml

Butter: 50g

Grated parmesan: 50g

Fresh thyme: 23 sprigs

Extra virgin olive oil: 2 tablespoons

Salt and Pepper To Taste

Preparation:

Clean and cut the strawberries into pieces. Finely chop the onion. In a saucepan, heat the vegetable broth. In another pan, heat the extra virgin olive oil, add the chopped onion and fry until translucent. Add the rice and toast it for a few minutes, then add the dry white wine and let the alcohol evaporate. Add a ladle of hot broth at a time to the rice, stirring constantly and adding more broth as it is absorbed. Halfway through cooking the rice (about 10 minutes), add the strawberries cut into pieces and continue cooking the risotto until it is al dente. At the end of cooking, mix the risotto with the butter, add the grated parmesan and the fresh thyme leaves. Adjust salt and pepper according to taste. Serve hot.

PASTA WITH APPLE SAUCE AND VEGETABLE SAUSAGE

Preparation Times: 10 minutes

Cooking Times: 20/25 minutes

Doses for 4 People

Ingredients:

Pasta to taste (penne, fusilli, or other short pasta): 400g

Rennet apples: 2

Vegetable sausage: 200g

Onion: 1

Cooking cream (vegetable if you prefer): 200ml

Extra virgin olive oil: 2 tablespoons

Salt and Pepper To Taste

Preparation:

Cut the apples and onion into cubes. In a pan, heat the extra virgin olive oil, add the chopped onion and brown it. Add the apples and cook until soft. Add the chopped vegetable sausage to the pan and brown. Add the cooking cream and cook over medium heat for a few minutes until the sauce thickens. In the meantime, cook the pasta in plenty of salted water following the instructions on the package. Drain it al dente and add it to the sauce in the pan. Mix the pasta well with the sauce and sauté for a minute over medium-high heat to blend the flavors. Serve hot, possibly adding freshly ground pepper as a finishing touch.

BROWN RICE SALAD WITH MANGO AND AVOCADO

Preparation Times: 15/20 minutes

Cooking times: 30/40 minutes

Doses for 4 People

Ingredients:

Brown rice: 300g

Ripe mango: 1

Ripe avocado: 2

Red onion: 1

Lime juice: 2 tablespoons

Fresh coriander: 1 bunch

Extra virgin olive oil: 3 tablespoons

Salt and Pepper To Taste

Preparation:

Cook brown rice in boiling salted water
following package instructions. Drain it al
dente and let it cool. Dice the mango,
avocado and red onion. Finely chop the fresh
coriander. In a large bowl, combine the
cooled brown rice, mango, avocado, red
onion and fresh cilantro. Add the lime juice,
extra virgin olive oil, salt and pepper. Gently
mix all the ingredients so as not to crush the
avocado too much. Let the salad rest in the
refrigerator for about 30 minutes before
serving to let the flavors blend.

LINGUINE WITH AVOCADO CREAM AND CHERRY TOMATOES

Preparation Times: 15/20 minutes

Cooking Times: 10/12 minutes

Doses for 4 People

Ingredients:

Linguine: 400g

Ripe avocado: 2

Cherry tomatoes: 250g

Garlic: 2 cloves

Fresh basil: 1 bunch

Extra virgin olive oil: 4 tablespoons

Salt and Pepper To Taste

Preparation:

Cook the linguine in boiling salted water following the instructions on the package. Drain them al dente and keep them aside. In the meantime, prepare the avocado cream: peel and remove the stone from the avocados, put them in a blender adding a clove of garlic, fresh basil, extra virgin olive oil, salt and pepper. Blend until you obtain a smooth cream. Cut the cherry tomatoes in half and finely chop the other clove of garlic. In a pan, heat a little extra virgin olive oil, add the chopped garlic and brown it lightly. Add the cherry tomatoes and cook for a few minutes until they start to release their juices. Add the drained linguine to the pan with the cherry tomatoes, add the prepared avocado cream and mix well to blend all the flavours. Serve the linguine with a sprinkling of freshly ground black pepper and, if desired, basil leaves as a garnish.

RECIPES
SECOND DISHES

BAKED SALMON WITH AROMATIC HERB CRUST

Preparation Times: 10/15 minutes

Cooking times: 15/20 minutes

Doses for 4 People

Ingredients:

Salmon fillets: 4

(about 150g each)

Grated bread: 100g

Fresh aromatic herbs

chopped (parsley,

thyme, rosemary, oregano): 3 tablespoons

Garlic: 2 cloves, finely chopped

Grated lemon zest: from 1 lemon

Salt and Pepper To Taste

Extra virgin olive oil: 4 tablespoons

Preparation:

Preheat the oven to 180°C. In a bowl, mix the breadcrumbs, chopped aromatic herbs, garlic, grated lemon zest, salt, pepper and extra virgin olive oil. Place the salmon fillets on a baking tray lined with baking paper. Spread the herb crust evenly over the salmon fillets, pressing it gently with your hands to help it stick. Bake in a preheated oven for about 15/20 minutes or until the salmon is cooked and the crust is golden and crunchy. Serve hot accompanied by lemon slices if desired.

SEA BASS FILLET IN PAPER WITH VEGETABLES

Preparation Times: 15/20 minutes

Cooking Times: 20/25 minutes

Doses for 4 People

Ingredients:

Sea bass fillets: 4

Courgettes: 2, cut into thin rounds

Cherry tomatoes: 200g, cut in half

Red onion: 1, thinly sliced

Fresh parsley: 1 bunch, chopped

Salt and Pepper To Taste

Aluminum foil

Preparation:

Preheat the oven to 180°C. Divide the sea bass fillets into 4 portions and place each portion on aluminum foil large enough to wrap the fish. Distribute the courgettes, cherry tomatoes and onion slices on each sea bass fillet. Sprinkle fresh chopped parsley over the fish and vegetables. Add salt and pepper to taste. Close the aluminum foil to form well-sealed packages. Place the packets on a baking tray and cook in the preheated oven for about 20/25 minutes or until the sea bass and vegetables are cooked. Open the packages carefully (watch out for steam) and serve hot directly in aluminum foil to maintain the heat.

GRILLED TUNA WITH CITRUS SAUCE

Preparation Times: 15/20 minutes

Cooking times: 6/8 minutes

Doses for 4 People

Ingredients:

Fresh tuna fillets:

4 (approximately 150g each)

Grated lemon and orange zest:

from 1 lemon and 1 orange

Lemon and orange juice:

from 1 lemon and 1 orange

Extra virgin olive oil: 4 tablespoons

Garlic: 2 cloves, finely chopped

Fresh parsley: 2 tablespoons, chopped

Salt and Pepper To Taste

Preparation:

Preheat grill to medium high heat. In a bowl, mix together the grated lemon and orange zest, the lemon and orange juice, the extra virgin olive oil, the chopped garlic, the fresh parsley, salt and pepper. Brush the tuna fillets with the prepared marinade and leave them to marinate for approximately 1015 minutes. Grill the tuna fillets for 34 minutes per side, or until cooked through but still slightly pink inside. While the tuna is grilling, you can heat the remaining marinade in a small saucepan until it reduces and becomes a thick sauce. Serve the grilled tuna with the prepared citrus sauce.

SHRIMP AND MIXED VEGETABLE SKEWERS

Preparation Times: 20/25 minutes (marinade included)

Cooking Times: 810 minutes

Doses for 4 People

Ingredients:

Fresh shelled prawns: 1620

Peppers of various colors: 2, cut into cubes

Red onion: 1, chopped

Courgettes: 2, cut into rounds

Lemon juice: from 1 lemon

Extra virgin olive oil: 4 tablespoons

Garlic: 2 cloves, finely chopped

Salt and Pepper To Taste

Skewer sticks (wood or metal)

Preparation:

In a bowl, mix together the lemon juice, extra virgin olive oil, minced garlic, salt and pepper. Place the prawns in the prepared marinade and leave them to marinate in the refrigerator for about 15/20 minutes. Weave the peppers, onion and courgettes onto the skewer sticks, alternating them with the marinated prawns. Preheat grill to medium-high heat. Cook the skewers on the hot grill for 34 minutes per side, or until the prawns are cooked through and the vegetables are lightly browned. Serve the skewers hot with a squeeze of fresh lemon juice, if desired.

CHICKEN BREAST WITH LEMON AND ASPARAGUS

Preparation Times: 10/15 minutes

Cooking Times: 20/25 minutes

Doses for 4 People

Ingredients:

Chicken Breast: 4 fillets

Asparagus: 1 bunch, hard parts removed

Lemon juice: from 2 lemons

Grated lemon zest: from 1 lemon

Garlic: 3 cloves, finely chopped

Fresh thyme: 2 tablespoons, chopped

Extra virgin olive oil: 4 tablespoons

Salt and Pepper To Taste

Preparation:

Preheat the oven to 200°C. In a bowl, mix together the lemon juice, grated lemon zest, minced garlic, fresh thyme, salt, pepper and extra virgin olive oil. Arrange the chicken breast fillets and asparagus on a baking tray. Pour the prepared marinade over the top, making sure to evenly cover the chicken and asparagus. Cook in the preheated oven for about 20/25 minutes or until the chicken is cooked and the asparagus is tender. Once cooked, you can serve the chicken breast with hot asparagus.

BAKED TURKEY WITH POTATOES AND ROSEMARY

Preparation Times: 20/25 minutes (marinade included)

Cooking Times: 1 hour and 15 minutes

Doses for 4 People

Ingredients:

Turkey fillet: 800g

1kg Potatoes: 4 medium, cut into thick slices

Fresh rosemary: 34 sprigs

Garlic: 3 cloves, finely chopped

Extra virgin olive oil: 4 tablespoons

Lemon juice: from 1 lemon

Salt and Pepper To Taste

Preparation:

In a bowl, mix the extra virgin olive oil, lemon juice, chopped garlic, salt, pepper and fresh rosemary. Marinate the turkey fillet with this mixture for at least 15/20 minutes. Preheat the oven to 180°C. Arrange the potato slices on a baking tray and place the marinated turkey fillet on top. Place in the oven and cook for about 1 hour 1 hour and 15 minutes, or until the turkey is golden brown and the potatoes are soft. Let it rest for a few minutes before cutting the turkey into slices and serving with the potatoes.

ROAST DUCK BREAST WITH RED FRUIT SAUCE

Preparation Times: 15/20 minutes (marinade included)

Cooking Times: 20/25 minutes

Doses for 4 People

Ingredients:

Duck Breast: 4 fillets

Red fruits (strawberries, raspberries, blueberries): 200g

Balsamic vinegar: 2 tablespoons

Brown sugar: 2 tablespoons

Red wine: 1/2 cup

Beef broth: 1/2 cup

Fresh rosemary: 2 sprigs

Salt and Pepper To Taste

Preparation:

Preheat the oven to 200°C. Lightly score the skin of the duck fillets, avoiding cutting the meat. Season with salt and pepper and leave to marinate for at least 15/20 minutes. Heat the balsamic vinegar and brown sugar in a pan until the sugar has dissolved. Add the red fruits and cook for a few minutes until the fruits begin to release their juices. Add the red wine and beef broth and let the sauce reduce until it is slightly thick. In a hot non-stick pan, place the duck breast fillets skin side down and cook for 3/4 minutes per side to get medium doneness or to your liking. Bake the duck fillets in the preheated oven for about 5/7 minutes or until cooked to your liking. Once cooked, serve the duck breast fillets hot accompanied by the prepared red fruit sauce.

VEAL SCALLOPS WITH MARSALA WITH MUSHROOMS

Preparation Times: 20/25 minutes

Cooking times: 15/20 minutes

Doses for 4 People

Ingredients:

Veal scallops: 8

Champignon mushrooms: 250g, cut into slices

Marsala: 1 cup

Beef broth: 1/2 cup

Flour: 3 tablespoons

Butter: 4 tablespoons

Extra virgin olive oil: 2 tablespoons

Fresh parsley: 2 tablespoons, chopped

Salt and Pepper To Taste

Preparation:

In a skillet, heat the extra-virgin olive oil and 2 tablespoons butter over medium-high heat. Lightly coat the scallops in the flour and then place them in the hot pan, cook them for 2/3 minutes on each side until they are golden. Remove the scallops from the pan and set aside. In the same pan, add 2 tablespoons butter and cook the mushrooms until soft and golden. Add the Marsala and the meat broth. Let it cook until the sauce has thickened slightly. Take the scallops and put them back in the pan with the mushroom and Marsala sauce, leaving to flavor for another 5 minutes over medium/low heat. Add the chopped fresh parsley and mix well. Serve the scallops hot with the mushroom sauce on top.

TOFU SAUTEED WITH VEGETABLES IN THE WOK

Preparation Times: 15/20 minutes

Cooking Times: 10/15 minutes

Doses for 4 People

Ingredients:

Tofu: 400g, drained and cut into cubes

Mixed vegetables of your choice (peppers, carrots,

courgettes, onions, broccoli): 500g,

cut into julienne or cubes

Soy sauce: 3 tablespoons

Sesame oil: 2 tablespoons

Garlic: 2 cloves, finely chopped

Fresh ginger: 1 tablespoon, grated

Toasted sesame seeds: 1 tablespoon
(optional)

Salt and pepper:

Preparation:

In a skillet or wok, heat the sesame oil over
medium-high heat. Add the garlic and grated
ginger, fry for about 1 minute or until
fragrant. Add the diced tofu and sauté until
they are golden on all sides, it will take about
5/7 minutes. Add the julienned or diced
vegetables and continue to sauté everything
for another 5/8 minutes until the vegetables
are cooked but still crunchy. Pour in the soy
sauce, mix well and make sure all the
ingredients are well seasoned. If desired, add
toasted sesame seeds to the top of the dish
before serving.

PAN-FED SEITAN WITH PEPPERS AND ONIONS

Preparation Times: 15/20 minutes

Cooking Times: 10/15 minutes

Doses for 4 People

Ingredients:

Seitan: 400g, cut into thin slices

Peppers of various colors: 2, cut into strips

Onions: 2 medium, thinly sliced

Garlic: 2 cloves, finely chopped

Extra virgin olive oil: 3 tablespoons

Soy sauce: 2 tablespoons

Paprika: 1 tsp

Black pepper: to taste

Fresh parsley: 2 tablespoons, chopped (optional)

Salt to taste

Preparation:

In a large skillet, heat the extra virgin olive oil over medium-high heat. Add the minced garlic and fry for about 1 minute or until golden and fragrant. Add the seitan slices and brown them for 3/5 minutes until they are lightly golden. Add the striped onions and peppers to the pan. Continue cooking for another 5 to 8 minutes or until the vegetables are cooked but still crunchy. Add soy sauce, paprika, black pepper and mix well. Add salt if necessary and, if desired, sprinkle fresh chopped parsley over the dish before serving.

BAKED TOFU WITH TOMATO AND BASIL SAUCE

Preparation Times: 20/25 minutes

Cooking times: 25/30 minutes

Doses for 4 People

Ingredients:

Tofu: 500g, drained and

cut into thick slices

Diced tomatoes: 400g

(canned or fresh)

Garlic: 3 cloves, finely chopped

Fresh basil: 1 bunch, chopped

Extra virgin olive oil: 3 tablespoons

Salt and pepper:

Preparation:

Preheat the oven to 180°C. In a bowl, mix the diced tomatoes with the chopped garlic, fresh basil, salt, pepper and two tablespoons of extra virgin olive oil. Place the tofu slices on a baking tray lightly greased with oil. Pour the prepared tomato sauce over the top, making sure to cover the tofu evenly. Bake the tofu in the preheated oven for about 25/30 minutes or until the sauce has thickened slightly and the tofu is golden. Once cooked, serve the baked tofu with the tomato and basil sauce on top.

SEITAN IN SWEET AND SOUR SAUCE WITH BASMATI RICE

Preparation Times: 20/25 minutes

Cooking times: 15/20 minutes

Doses for 4 People

Ingredients:

Seitan: 400g, cut into cubes or slices

Basmati rice: 300g

Peppers of various colors: 2, cut into strips

Onion: 1 large, thinly sliced

Apple cider vinegar: 3 tablespoons

Brown sugar: 2 tablespoons

Soy sauce: 2 tablespoons

Extra virgin olive oil: 3 tablespoons

Fresh ginger: 1 tablespoon, grated

Garlic: 2 cloves, finely chopped

Black pepper: to taste Salt: to taste

Preparation:

Cook the basmati rice according to the package instructions and set aside. In a pan, heat the extra virgin olive oil over medium-high heat. Add minced garlic, grated ginger, striped peppers and sliced onions. Fry for about 3/5 minutes or until the vegetables are soft. Add the diced seitan and let it cook for another 5/7 minutes until it is lightly golden. In a separate bowl, mix the apple cider vinegar, brown sugar, soy sauce, a pinch of salt and black pepper. Pour sweet and sour sauce mixture over seitan and pan-fried vegetables. Leave to cook for another 35 minutes until the sauce has thickened slightly and the seitan is well cooked. Serve the seitan in sweet and sour sauce over the previously prepared basmati rice.

GRILLED BEEF STEAK WITH VEGETABLE SIDE SIDE

Preparation Times: 10/15 minutes (marinade included)

Cooking Times: 10/15 minutes

Doses for 2 People

Ingredients:

Beef Steak: 2 pieces (250g each)

Courgettes: 2, cut into long slices

Peppers of various colors: 2, cut into strips

Eggplant: 1, sliced

Tomatoes: 2, cut in half

Extra virgin olive oil: 3 tablespoons

Garlic: 2 cloves, finely chopped

Fresh rosemary: 2 sprigs

Salt and Pepper To Taste

Preparation:

Preheat grill or grill pan to medium-high heat. Season the beef steaks with extra virgin olive oil, minced garlic, fresh rosemary, salt and pepper. Let them marinate for about 10/15 minutes. Grill steaks for 35 minutes per side (depending on desired thickness and preferred doneness). In the meantime, brush the vegetables (courgettes, peppers, aubergines and tomatoes) with oil. Place the vegetables on the grill and cook them for about 3/5 minutes per side, until they are well marked and tender. Once cooked, serve the grilled beef steaks with vegetables as a side dish.

BEEF STEW WITH SWEET POTATOES

Preparation Times: 20/25 minutes

Cooking times: 1 hour

Doses for 4 People

Ingredients:

Beef for Stew:

800g cut into cubes

Sweet Potatoes: 3 medium, cut into cubes

Onion: 1 large, finely chopped

Garlic: 3 cloves, finely chopped

Beef broth: 2 cups

Diced tomatoes: 1 can (400g)

Extra virgin olive oil: 3 tablespoons

Fresh rosemary: 2 sprigs

Salt and Pepper To Taste

Preparation:

In a large pot, heat the extra virgin olive oil over medium-high heat. Add the chopped onion and garlic and fry for 2/3 minutes until golden. Add the diced beef and brown until browned on all sides. Add diced sweet potatoes, diced tomatoes, beef broth, fresh rosemary, salt and pepper. Bring everything to the boil, then reduce the heat and leave to simmer for about 1 hour 1 hour and 15 minutes or until the meat and potatoes are tender. Once ready, serve the beef stew with sweet potatoes piping hot.

PORK FILLET WITH APPLE SAUCE AND CINNAMON

Preparation Times: 15/20 minutes (marinade included)

Cooking Times: 20/25 minutes

Doses for 4 People

Ingredients:

Pork fillet: 4 pieces (200g each)

Apples: 2 large, peeled and cut into slices

Onion: 1 medium, thinly sliced

Ground cinnamon: 1 teaspoon

Butter: 3 tablespoons

Beef broth: 1/2 cup

Salt and Pepper To Taste

Preparation:

Preheat the oven to 180°C. Season the pork fillets with salt, pepper and ground cinnamon. Let them marinate for about 10/15 minutes. In a skillet, melt the butter over medium-high heat. Add the pork slices and brown them for 2/3 minutes on each side until they are golden brown. Remove the pork from the pan and place it on a baking tray. In the same pan, add the apple slices and onion slices. Cook for 3/5 minutes until soft and lightly golden. Add the beef broth to the pan and mix well. Pour this mixture over the pork tenderloins in the baking dish. Bake in the preheated oven for about 15/20 minutes or until the pork is completely cooked and the apples are soft and caramelized. Once cooked, serve the pork tenderloin with the apples and cinnamon sauce on top.

ROAST TURKEY WITH AROMATIC HERBS

Preparation Times: 20/25 minutes (marinade included)

Cooking times: 1 hour

Doses for 46 People

Ingredients:

Turkey breasts: 1.5 kg

Fresh rosemary: 2 sprigs

Fresh sage: 4 leaves

Fresh thyme: 2 sprigs

Garlic: 4 cloves, crushed

Lemon juice: 3 tablespoons

Extra virgin olive oil: 4 tablespoons

Salt and Pepper To Taste

Preparation:

Preheat the oven to 180°C. In a bowl, mix the extra virgin olive oil with the lemon juice, the aromatic herbs (rosemary, sage, thyme), the crushed garlic cloves, salt and pepper. Massage this marinade onto the turkey breast and leave to marinate for at least 15/20 minutes. Place the turkey on a baking tray and bake in the preheated oven. Cook for approximately 1 hour 1 hour and 15 minutes or until the turkey has reached an internal temperature of 165°F. Once cooked, let the turkey rest for a few minutes before slicing and serving.

OMELETTE WITH MIXED MUSHROOMS AND PARSLEY

Preparation Times: 10/15 minutes

Cooking times: 15/20 minutes

Doses for 4 People

Ingredients: Eggs: 8 large

Mixed mushrooms (porcini, champignons, pleurotus): 400g, cleaned and cut into slices

Onion: 1 medium, finely chopped

Fresh parsley: 2 tablespoons, chopped

Grated cheese (parmesan or pecorino): 4 tablespoons

Extra virgin olive oil: 2 tablespoons

Salt and Pepper To Taste

Preparation:

n a non-stick pan, heat the extra virgin olive oil over medium heat. Add chopped onions and mushrooms. Cook for 5/7 minutes until the mushrooms are golden and the water has evaporated. Drain off any excess liquid. In a bowl, beat the eggs with the grated cheese, chopped fresh parsley, salt and pepper. Add the mushrooms and onions to the bowl with the beaten eggs. Mix everything well. Heat another non-stick pan, lightly greased with oil or butter. Pour in the egg and mushroom mixture. Cook the omelette over medium-low heat for about 10/15 minutes or until it is well set. You can cover the pan with a lid to help even cooking. Once cooked on both sides, transfer the omelette to a serving plate and cut it into wedges to serve.

COOKED EGGS IN WITH SPINACH AND CHEESE

Preparation Times: 15/20 minutes

Cooking times: 15/20 minutes

Doses for 4 People

Ingredients:

Eggs: 8 medium

Fresh spinach: 400g, washed and cut into strips

Cheese to taste (e.g. cheese gruyère, cheddar, mozzarella):

100g, diced or grated

Cooking cream: 6 tablespoons

Butter: 1 tbsp

Nutmeg: to taste

Salt and Pepper To Taste

Preparation

Preheat the oven to 180°C. Lightly butter casseroles or small oven-safe bowls. Distribute the fresh spinach evenly in the casseroles. Add the grated or cubed cheese on top of the spinach. Add 1 tablespoon of heavy cream to each cocotte on top of the cheese. Break an egg for each cocotte without breaking the yolk. Add a pinch of salt, pepper and nutmeg to each egg. Place the cocottes in a baking tray and pour a little hot water into the pan around the cocottes. Bake the cocottes in the preheated oven for about 15/20 minutes or until the egg whites are solid and the yolks have the desired consistency. Once ready, serve the eggs in hot cocottes accompanied by toasted or crunchy bread for dipping.

OMELETTE WITH TOMATOES AND FRESH BASIL

Preparation Times: 10/15 minutes

Cooking Times: 5/7 minutes

Doses for 4 People

Ingredients:

Eggs: 6 large

Cherry tomatoes: 8, cut in half

Fresh basil: 8 leaves,

cut into thin strips

Cheese to taste (e.g. mozzarella,

fresh cheese): 50g, cut

diced or grated

Extra virgin olive oil: 1 tablespoon

Salt and Pepper To Taste

Preparation:

In a bowl, beat the eggs with a pinch of salt and pepper. Heat the extra virgin olive oil in a non-stick pan over medium heat. Pour the beaten eggs into the hot pan. When the edge of the omelette starts to set, add the halved cherry tomatoes, fresh basil and cheese on top of one half of the omelet. Using a spatula, fold the other half of the omelet over the filling and cook for another 1/2 minute until the cheese has melted and the omelette is golden. Using the spatula, transfer the omelette to a plate and serve hot.

SCRAMBLED EGGS WITH ASPARAGUS AND LIGHT BACON

Preparation Times: 10/15 minutes

Cooking Times: 10/12 minutes

Doses for 4 People

Ingredients:

Eggs: 8 medium

Asparagus: 20 stalks, cut into small pieces

Light or smoked bacon:

100 g, cut into cubes

Cheese to taste (e.g. pecorino,

parmesan): 50g, grated

Butter: 1 tbsp

Milk: 2 tablespoons

Salt and pepper:

Preparation:

In a pan, brown the bacon over medium heat until golden. Add the cut asparagus and cook for 5/7 minutes until tender. Keep aside. In a bowl, beat the eggs with the milk, a pinch of salt and pepper. Heat the butter in a nonstick pan over medium heat. Pour the beaten eggs into the hot pan. As the eggs begin to set, add the bacon and asparagus over the top of the eggs. Continue to gently mix the eggs until they take on a creamy consistency. Add the grated cheese on top of the scrambled eggs and mix quickly. Serve hot scrambled eggs accompanied by toasted or crunchy bread.

QUINOA AND BEANS BURGER WITH VEGETABLE SIDE DISH

Preparation Times: 20 minutes

Cooking Times: 25 minutes

Doses for 4 People

Ingredients:

Quinoa: 1 cup, already cooked

Black beans: 400g, drained and rinsed

Onion: 1 medium, finely chopped

Breadcrumbs: ½ cup

Egg: 1 large

Paprika: 1 tsp

Cumin powder: 1 teaspoon

Salt and Pepper To Taste

Hamburger bread: 4 pieces

Lettuce, tomato,

sliced cucumbers for garnish

Preparation:

In a large bowl, mash the cooked black beans and add the quinoa, chopped onion, breadcrumbs, egg, paprika, cumin powder, salt and pepper. Mix well until you obtain a homogeneous mixture. Form four burgers from the mixture obtained. Heat a nonstick pan over medium heat. Cook the quinoa and bean burgers for 5 minutes per side or until golden brown. Lightly toast the hamburger buns. Assemble the quinoa and bean burgers on toasted buns and garnish with lettuce leaves, tomato slices and cucumber. Serve hot.

BAKED VEGETABLE CASSEROLE WITH SWEET POTATOES

Preparation Times: 20/25 minutes

Cooking times: 35/40 minutes

Doses for 46 People

Ingredients:

Sweet potatoes: 3 medium, peeled

and cut into thin slices

Courgettes: 2 medium, cut into thin slices

Eggplant: 1 large, thinly sliced

Tomatoes: 34 large, cut into slices

Mozzarella or cheese of your choice: 200g,
cut into cubes

Fresh basil: a few leaves

Extra virgin olive oil: 3 tablespoons

Salt and Pepper To Taste

Preparation:

Preheat the oven to 180°C. On a baking sheet, arrange a layer of sweet potato slices, followed by a layer of zucchini, eggplant, and tomato slices. Add salt, pepper and basil leaves between the layers of vegetables. Repeat the same process until all the vegetables are used up. Bake the vegetable casserole for about 35/40 minutes or until the vegetables are soft and lightly golden on the surface. A few minutes after cooking, add the cubes of mozzarella or other cheese to the casserole and cook au gratin until the cheese is melted and lightly golden. Once cooked, serve the baked vegetable casserole as a side dish.

LENTIL AND SWEET POTATO CURRY

Preparation Times: 15/20 minutes

Cooking Times: 30/35 minutes

Doses for 4 People

Ingredients:

Red Lentils: 1 cup, rinsed

Sweet potatoes: 2 medium,

peeled and cut into cubes

Onion: 1 large, finely chopped

Garlic: 2 cloves, minced

Fresh ginger: 1 teaspoon, grated

Curry powder: 2/3 teaspoons

Coconut milk: 1 can (400 ml)

Vegetable broth: 2 cups

Extra virgin olive oil: 2 tablespoons

Salt and Pepper To Taste

Fresh coriander or parsley

for garnish (optional)

Preparation:

In a large pot, heat the extra virgin olive oil over medium heat. Add the onion, garlic and ginger and cook for 2/3 minutes until golden. Add the curry powder and stir for a minute. Add the diced sweet potatoes, rinsed red lentils, coconut milk and vegetable broth. Bring everything to the boil. Reduce the heat and leave to cook over medium-low heat for 25/30 minutes or until the potatoes and lentils are soft and the curry has reached the desired consistency. Add salt and pepper to your taste. Serve the lentil and sweet potato curry hot, garnished with fresh coriander or parsley if desired. You can serve it with basmati rice or naan bread.

VEGAN BEAN AND QUINOA MEATBALLS

Preparation Times: 20/25 minutes

Cooking Times: 20/25 minutes

Doses for 4 People

Ingredients:

Black beans: 400g, drained and rinsed

Cooked quinoa: 1 cup

Onion: 1 medium, finely chopped

Garlic: 2 cloves, minced Breadcrumbs: ½ cup, Fresh parsley: 2 tablespoons, chopped

Paprika: 1 teaspoon Salt and pepper: to taste

Cumin powder: 1 teaspoon

Extra virgin olive oil: 2 tablespoons

Preparation:

Preheat the oven to 180°C and line a baking tray with baking paper.

In a bowl, coarsely mash the cooked black beans. Add the cooked quinoa, chopped onion, garlic, breadcrumbs, fresh parsley, paprika, cumin powder, salt and pepper to the mashed beans. Mix well until you obtain a homogeneous mixture. Form meatballs with the mixture and place them on the baking tray lined with baking paper. Cook in the preheated oven for 20/25 minutes or until the meatballs are golden. Once ready, serve the vegan bean and quinoa meatballs hot, accompanying them with a sauce of your choice or a vegan accompanying sauce. Preparation for the Tomato Sauce: In a skillet, heat the olive oil over medium heat. Add the onion and garlic, and sauté slightly. Add the peeled tomatoes and basil. Let it cook over medium-low heat for about 10/15 minutes until the sauce has thickened. Season with salt and pepper to taste. Pour the tomato sauce over the lentil meatballs before serving.

BAKED TURKEY WITH AROMATIC HERBS

Preparation Times: 15 minutes

Cooking times: 1 hour and 30 minutes

Doses for 46 People

Ingredients:

Turkey breast: 1, whole

Fresh rosemary: a few sprigs

Fresh sage: a few leaves

Fresh thyme: a few leaves

Garlic: 45 cloves, minced

Butter: 50g, at room temperature

Olive oil: 23 tablespoons

Salt and Pepper To Taste

Preparation:

Preheat the oven to 180°C. In a bowl, mix room temperature butter with minced garlic and fresh herbs. Season the turkey breast with salt and pepper. Gently lift the skin of the turkey and spread the butter and herb mixture under the skin, massaging well. Brush the surface of the turkey with a little olive oil. Place the turkey breast on a baking tray and cook for approximately 1 hour and 30 minutes or until the internal temperature reaches 75/80°C and the surface is golden. Let rest for a few minutes before slicing the turkey and serving.

SIDE DISH RECIPES

SPRING QUINOA SALAD

Preparation time: 30 minutes

Cooking time: 20 minutes

Doses: 4 people

Ingredients:

For the quinoa:

150 g of quinoa

300 ml of water

1/2 teaspoon salt

1 tablespoon extra virgin olive oil

For the vegetables:

200 g of asparagus, 150 g of peas

100 g of carrots, 1 courgette

For the lemon yogurt sauce:

150 g of Greek yogurt

1 tablespoon lemon juice

1/2 teaspoon Dijon mustard

1/4 teaspoon salt, Pepper to taste

1 tablespoon chopped fresh herbs

(basil, mint, chives)

To garnish: Sesame seeds

Fresh mint leaves

Preparation:

Cook the quinoa: rinse the quinoa under running water. In a saucepan, combine the quinoa, water and salt. Bring to the boil, cover with a lid and cook over low heat for about 15 minutes, until the water is completely absorbed. Remove from the heat and let rest for 5 minutes. Prepare the vegetables: wash and clean the vegetables. Cut the asparagus into small pieces, shell the peas, carrots and courgette into thin slices. Steam vegetables:

Steam vegetables for about 5-10 minutes, until, tender but still crunchy. Make the lemon yogurt sauce: In a bowl, mix the Greek yogurt, lemon juice, Dijon mustard, salt, pepper, and chopped fresh herbs. Assemble the salad: In a large bowl, combine the cooked quinoa, steamed vegetables and lemon yogurt dressing. Stir gently to combine the ingredients. Garnish: decorate with sesame seeds and fresh mint leaves. Serve: Serve the salad at room temperature or warm.

STEAMED VEGETABLES WITH LEMON YOGURT SAUCE

Preparation time: 20 minutes

Cooking time: 10 minutes

Doses: 4 people

Ingredients:

For the vegetables:

200 g of mixed vegetables

(choice of broccoli, cauliflower,

carrots, green beans, courgettes)

For the lemon yogurt sauce:

150 g of Greek yogurt

1 tablespoon lemon juice

1/2 teaspoon Dijon mustard

1/4 teaspoon salt

Pepper as needed

1 tablespoon chopped fresh herbs

(basil, mint, chives)

Preparation:

Steam vegetables: wash and clean the vegetables. Cut them into similar sized pieces. Steam the vegetables for about 5-10 minutes, until they are tender but still crunchy. Prepare the lemon yogurt sauce: in a bowl, mix the Greek yogurt, lemon juice, Dijon mustard, salt, pepper and chopped fresh herbs. Assemble the dish: arrange the steamed vegetables on a platter. Drizzle the vegetables with the lemon yogurt sauce. Serve: Serve the steamed vegetables with lemon yogurt sauce piping hot, as a side dish.

SPINACH SALAD WITH ALMONDS AND STRAWBERRIES

Preparation time: 15 minutes

Doses: 4 people

Ingredients:

200 g of fresh spinach

150 g of strawberries

50 g of toasted flaked almonds

50 g of crumbled feta

1 small red onion, finely chopped

1 tablespoon extra virgin olive oil

Lemon juice (to taste)

Salt and Pepper To Taste

Preparation:

Wash the spinach and strawberries thoroughly. Dry well with a kitchen towel. Cut the strawberries in half or quarters, depending on their size. In a large bowl, combine the spinach, strawberries, slivered almonds, crumbled feta and chopped onion. Season with extra virgin olive oil, lemon juice, salt and pepper to taste. Stir gently to combine the ingredients. Serve the spinach salad with almonds and strawberries immediately.

BAKED SWEET POTATOES WITH AROMATIC HERBS

Preparation time: 15 minutes

Cooking time: 45 minutes

Doses: 4 people

Ingredients:

4 sweet potatoes

2 tablespoons extra virgin olive oil

1 tablespoon of aromatic herbs chopped (rosemary, thyme, sage)

Salt and Pepper To Taste

Preparation:

Preheat the oven to 200°C. Wash and dry the sweet potatoes thoroughly. Peel the sweet potatoes (optional: you can also leave them in the skin for a higher fiber content) and cut them into cubes of about 2 cm. In a large bowl, combine the sweet potatoes, extra virgin olive oil, chopped herbs, salt and pepper to taste. Mix well to evenly distribute the seasoning. Place the sweet potatoes on a baking tray lined with baking paper. Bake in the oven for about 45 minutes, turning the potatoes halfway through cooking, until they are golden and crispy on the outside and soft on the inside. Serve the baked sweet potatoes with hot herbs as a side dish.

ROASTED CAULIFLOWER WITH TURMERIC AND PAPRIKA

Preparation time: 20 minutes

Cooking time: 40 minutes

Doses: 4 people

Ingredients:

1 medium cauliflower

2 tablespoons extra virgin olive oil

1 teaspoon turmeric powder

1/2 teaspoon sweet paprika

1/2 teaspoon salt

Pepper as needed

Preparation

Preheat the oven to 200°C. Cut the cauliflower into medium-sized florets. In a large bowl, combine the cauliflower florets, extra virgin olive oil, turmeric powder, sweet paprika, salt and pepper. Mix well to evenly distribute the seasoning. Arrange the cauliflower florets on a baking tray lined with baking paper. Bake in the oven for about 40 minutes, turning the florets halfway through cooking, until they are golden and crispy on the outside and soft on the inside. Serve the roasted cauliflower with turmeric and paprika hot as a side dish.

GRILLED COURGETTES WITH BASIL PESTO

Preparation time: 15 minutes

Cooking time: 10 minutes

Doses: 4 people

Ingredients:

2 medium courgettes

2 tablespoons extra virgin olive oil

Salt and Pepper To Taste

For the basil pesto:

50 g of fresh basil leaves

20 g of pine nuts

2 cloves of garlic

50 g of grated parmesan

100 ml of extra virgin olive oil

Salt to taste

Preparation

Wash and dry the courgettes carefully. Cut the courgettes into longitudinal slices about 1 cm thick. In a bowl, combine the courgettes, extra virgin olive oil, salt and pepper to taste. Mix well to evenly distribute the seasoning. Heat a grill or non-stick pan. Grill the courgettes for about 5 minutes per side, until golden and grilled. In the meantime, prepare the basil pesto: in a blender, combine the basil leaves, pine nuts, garlic cloves, grated Parmigiano Reggiano, extra virgin olive oil and salt. Blend until you obtain a creamy pesto. Arrange the grilled courgettes on a serving plate. Drizzle the courgettes with the basil pesto. Serve the grilled courgettes with basil pesto piping hot.

SAUTEED GREEN BEANS WITH GARLIC AND ALMONDS

Preparation time: 15 minutes

Cooking time: 10 minutes

Doses: 4 people

Ingredients:

250 g of green beans

2 tablespoons extra virgin olive oil

2 cloves garlic, finely chopped

50 g of flaked almonds

Salt and Pepper To Taste

Preparation:

Wash and trim the green beans. Boil the green beans in boiling salted water for about 5 minutes, until tender but still crunchy. Drain the green beans and let them cool. Heat the extra virgin olive oil in a pan. Saute the minced garlic for a minute, until golden. Add the boiled green beans and the sliced almonds. Stir-fry for a couple of minutes, stirring often, until the green beans are well seasoned and the almonds toasted. Serve the green beans sautéed with garlic and almonds hot as a side dish.

STEAMED ARTICHOKES WITH MUSTARD SAUCE AND HONEY

Preparation time: 20 minutes

Cooking time: 20 minutes

Doses: 4 people

Ingredients:

4 artichokes

1 lemon

2 tablespoons extra virgin olive oil

Salt and Pepper To Taste

For the mustard and honey sauce:

2 tablespoons Dijon mustard

2 tablespoons honey

1 tablespoon lemon juice

2 tablespoons extra virgin olive oil

Salt and Pepper To Taste

Preparation:

Clean the artichokes: remove the hard outer leaves, cut the stem and the tips of the thorns. Peel the artichokes with a sharp knife, being careful not to let them blacken. Immerse the cleaned artichokes in water acidulated with lemon juice to prevent them from blackening. Steam the artichokes for about 20 minutes, until they are tender. In the meantime, prepare the mustard and honey sauce: in a bowl, mix the Dijon mustard, honey, lemon juice, extra virgin olive oil olive, salt and pepper to taste. Drain the steamed artichokes. Arrange the artichokes on a serving plate. Drizzle the artichokes with the mustard and honey sauce. Serve the steamed artichokes with mustard sauce and honey piping hot as a side dish.

BAKED TOMATOES WITH BASIL AND FETA CHEESE

Preparation time: 15 minutes

Cooking time: 20 minutes

Doses: 4 people

Ingredients:

500 g of cherry tomatoes

2 tablespoons extra virgin olive oil

Salt and Pepper To Taste

100g crumbled feta

Chopped fresh basil (to taste)

Preparation:

Preheat the oven to 200°C. Wash and dry the cherry tomatoes. Arrange the cherry tomatoes on a baking tray lined with baking paper. Season the cherry tomatoes with extra virgin olive oil, salt and pepper to taste. Bake in the oven for about 20 minutes, until the cherry tomatoes are slightly wilted and golden. Remove the cherry tomatoes from the oven and sprinkle them with their cooking sauce. Add the crumbled feta and chopped fresh basil. Mix gently and serve the baked cherry tomatoes with basil and feta hot or at room temperature.

SAUTÉED MUSHROOMS WITH PARSLEY AND LEMON

Preparation time: 10 minutes

Cooking time: 15 minutes

Doses: 4 people

Ingredients:

400 g of mixed mushrooms (choice of mushrooms, porcini mushrooms, pleurotus)

2 tablespoons extra virgin olive oil

1 clove garlic, finely chopped

Salt and Pepper To Taste

Chopped fresh parsley (to taste)

Lemon juice (to taste)

Preparation:

Clean the mushrooms: cut them into slices or cubes, depending on their variety. Heat the extra virgin olive oil in a pan. Saute the minced garlic for a minute, until golden. Add the mushrooms and cook them for about 15 minutes, stirring often, until they are well browned and dry. Salt and pepper to taste. Add chopped fresh parsley and lemon juice to taste. Mix gently and serve the sautéed mushrooms with parsley and lemon piping hot, as a side dish.

CONCLUSION

Dear Reader, We come to the end of this journey towards Circadian Diet 2025. It has been an exciting journey, exploring the deep connections between our bodies, food, and the natural rhythm of our world. I hope you have found these pages full of inspiration, rich in knowledge and, above all, useful on your path to wellness. The 110 recipes shared on these pages have been selected with love and care to offer a variety of flavors and nutrients that align with the body's circadian rhythms. Each dish is designed not only to delight your palate, but also to support your health and internal balance. The fundamental message of this guide is not only to offer a series of recipes, but to invite you to rediscover the profound connection between what we put on our plate and how this affects our overall well-being. The circadian diet is more than a trend fleeting: it is an invitation to get closer to nature and the harmony of our body. I would love to hear your feedback on this trip. If the book has inspired you, helped you in any way, I would be infinitely grateful if you could take a moment to leave a review. We are happy to have accompanied you on this journey towards a personalized and healthy diet. We hope the recipes and information in this book have inspired you to make more conscious food choices and achieve your wellness goals. Your words could be a guiding light for other wellness seekers embarking on this path. I thank you deeply for choosing "Circadian Diet 2025" as your travel companion towards a healthier and more conscious life. With gratitude, Sincerely,

[KLARLOCK]